01836

POLYMER SCIENCE AND TECHNOLOGY
Volume 8

POLYMERS IN MEDICINE AND SURGERY

POLYMER SCIENCE AND TECHNOLOGY

Volume 1 • STRUCTURE AND PROPERTIES OF POLYMER FILMS
   Edited by Robert W. Lenz and Richard S. Stein • 1972

Volume 2 • WATER-SOLUBLE POLYMERS
   Edited by N. M. Bikales • 1973

Volume 3 • POLYMERS AND ECOLOGICAL PROBLEMS
   Edited by James Guillet • 1973

Volume 4• RECENT ADVANCES IN POLYMER BLENDS, GRAFTS, AND BLOCKS
   Edited by L. H. Sperling • 1974

Volume 5 • ADVANCES IN POLYMER FRICTION AND WEAR (Parts A and B)
   Edited by Lieng-Huang Lee • 1974

Volume 6 • PERMEABILITY OF PLASTIC FILMS AND COATINGS
   TO GASES, VAPORS, AND LIQUIDS
   Edited by Harold B. Hopfenberg • 1974

Volume 7 • BIOMEDICAL APPLICATIONS OF POLYMERS
   Edited by Harry P. Gregor • 1975

Volume 8 • POLYMERS IN MEDICINE AND SURGERY
   Edited by Richard L. Kronenthal, Zale Oser, and E. Martin • 1975

Volume 9 • ADHESION SCIENCE AND TECHNOLOGY (Parts A and B)
   Edited by Lieng-Huang Lee • 1975

A Continuation Order Plan is available for this series. A continuation order will bring delivery of each new volume immediately upon publication. Volumes are billed only upon actual shipment. For further information please contact the publisher.

POLYMER SCIENCE AND TECHNOLOGY
Volume 8

POLYMERS IN MEDICINE AND SURGERY

Edited by

Richard L. Kronenthal
Ethicon Inc.
Somerville, New Jersey

Zale Oser
Patient Care Division
Johnson and Johnson
New Brunswick, New Jersey

and

E. Martin
Ethicon Inc.
Somerville, New Jersey

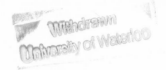
PLENUM PRESS · NEW YORK AND LONDON

Library of Congress Cataloging in Publication Data

Main entry under title:

Polymers in medicine and surgery.

   (Polymer science and technology; v. 8)
   "Proceedings of the Johnson & Johnson symposium held in Morristown, New Jersey, July 11-12, 1974."
   Includes bibliographical references.
   1. Polymers in medicine—Congresses. 2. Prosthesis—Congresses. I. Kronenthal, Richard L. II. Oser, Zale. III. Martin, E. IV. Johnson and Johnson, inc. V. Series. [DNLM: 1. Polymers—Congresses. 2. Biocompatible materials—Congresses. 3. Biomedical engineering—Congresses. QT34 P783 1974]

R857.P6P64	610'.28	75-33684

ISBN 0-306-36408-5

Proceedings of the Johnson & Johnson Symposium held in Morristown, New Jersey, July 11-12, 1974

© 1975 Plenum Press, New York
A Division of Plenum Publishing Corporation
227 West 17th Street, New York, N.Y. 10011

United Kingdom edition published by Plenum Press, London
A Division of Plenum Publishing Company, Ltd.
Davis House (4th Floor), 8 Scrubs Lane, Harlesden, London, NW10 6SE, England

Printed in the United States of America

HANS H. ZINSSER, M.D.

It was with deep regret that we learned of the untimely death of Hans Zinsser on August 14, 1974, less than five weeks after his participation in this Symposium.

Combining unusual abilities in both clinical medicine and the physical sciences, particularly electronics, Dr. Zinsser made important contributions to the study of pyelonephritis, kidney calculi and urological problems related to space medicine. He was a member of many scientific organizations including the New York Academy of Medicine, and the International Federation of Medical Electronics; he was a member of the advisory boards of the Institute of Radio Engineers and of the American Chemical Society, and was a member of the Associate Editorial Board of the New York State Journal of Medicine.

We keenly feel the loss we have all sustained and we will miss a distinguished scientist, clinician and good friend. This volume of contributions is dedicated to his memory.

PREFACE

The past decade has witnessed a vigorous growth in activities toward the development of a variety of biomedical devices ranging from the simple A-V shunt to the complex artificial heart. Research and development teams have been created comprising engineers, material scientists and clinicians and, perhaps for the first time, such groups are collaboratively bringing their respective talents to bear on problems associated with defects in the human organism. These collaborations have resulted in a proliferation of new information and a rapid and continuing redefinition of the frontiers of progress. It was to keep pace with these changes, and provide an updated view of the state of the art that this meeting was conceived.

The present volume marks the publication of the proceedings of the Johnson & Johnson Symposium held in Morristown, New Jersey, on July 11 and 12, 1974. It surveys the applications of polymers to medical and surgical problems and contains discussions on the biocompatibility of polymers, polymers as biomaterials, and the use of polymers in prosthetic devices and drug release systems. In addition, the Symposium offers recent perspectives on the critical problems of the material-tissue interface, the design criteria for silicone-based systems, and the varied use of polymers in artificial hearts, kidneys, eyes and lungs.

This Symposium was designed to provide an atmosphere for a stimulating and productive discussion among scientists and clinicians in the fields of biomaterials, biomedical engineering, pharmacology, urology, ophthalmology, orthopedics, pulmonary and cardiovascular diseases, and biomedical device development. It is hoped that researchers who were unable to attend the meeting will benefit by reviewing the proceedings.

The editors are particularly indebted to Dr. John Da Vanzo, Dr. Jacob Struck, Jr., Mr. Frank Servas and Dr. Douglas Walkling whose collaboration in organizing the Symposium was invaluable and to Mrs. Carol Volpi who skillfully, cheerfully and sometimes tearfully typed the manuscript.

Finally, the sponsorship of the Symposium by the Johnson & Johnson Council of Research Directors and, in particular, the inspired guidance of Mr. Foster B. Whitlock, Vice Chairman of the Board of Directors, Johnson & Johnson, and Dr. Charles Artandi, Vice President of Research, Ethicon, Inc., is gratefully acknowledged.

Richard L. Kronenthal
Zale Oser
E. Martin

August, 1975

CONTENTS

ARTIFICIAL ORGANS AND THEIR IMPACT

W. J. Kolff

Division of Artificial Organs, Department of Surgery, and The Institute for Biomedical Engineering, University of Utah, Salt Lake City, Utah 84112

ARTIFICIAL KIDNEYS

While artificial kidneys are being applied to 40, 000 people throughout the world, the search for the molecules most responsible for the clinical picture of uremia goes on. We have always held that uremia is not due to a single toxin but to the summation of all the substances retained in kidney failure and other factors that occur as well.

Although we do not wish to blame any particular molecule, Dr. Scribner in Seattle has some reason to believe that middle sized molecules, or "midi" molecules may be important for the distressing symptoms of neuropathy in patients sustained with artificial kidneys. The peritoneal membrane, being more permeable than most cellophanes, is effective in removing these molecules (see later). A very promising way to remove larger molecules is with charcoal.

Charcoal Artificial Kidney. Our Drs. Andrade and Lentz have coated carefully washed activated carbon (charcoal) with Hydron (Fig. 1). Hydron is the material that is used in soft contact lenses. Dr. Andrade can now flow blood directly over this charcoal. The charcoal retains its capacity to adsorb molecules on its surface but it does very little, if any damage to the blood cells and platelets. Charcoal artificial kidneys will do best what the cellophane or usual artificial kidneys do the least well, that is, the removal of

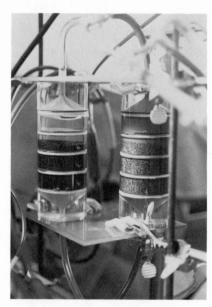

FIGURE 1. Charcoal artificial kidney. The charcoal is coated
with Hydron-like material to make it more blood-compatible
(Andrade and Lentz).

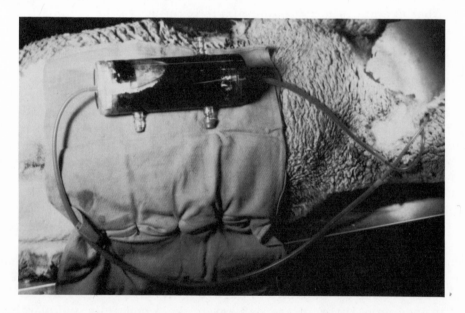

FIGURE 2. Preliminary model of WAK in blood circulation of
sheep (Dharnidharka).

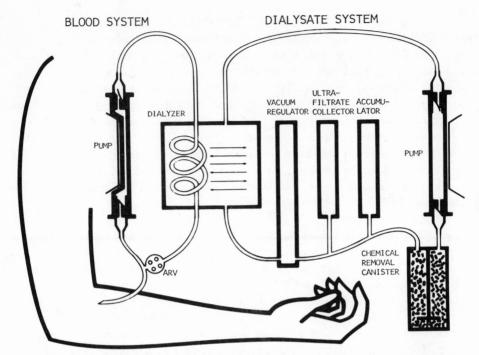

FIGURE 3. Diagram of wearable artificial kidney; single needle
system (Jacobsen).

the middle and large molecules. A combination of the two techniques therefore seems to be promising.

     Wearable Artificial Kidney.* Dr. S. Dharnidharka has done
some interesting experiments (Fig. 2). If a capillary kidney is
used and one sucks with an ordinary syringe, a partial vacuum
(300 ml of mercury) is created on the outside and ultrafiltrate
forms at the rate of 340 cc per hour which then can be used instead
of regular dialyzing fluid. Elimination of dialyzing fluid is of
course wonderful because it not only makes the artificial kidney
much smaller, but it also eliminates all the dangers connected with
the use of tap water. To remove the retention products, the ultrafiltrate must now be circulated over charcoal and other adsorbents.

*Our work on the wearable artificial kidney is supported by
  Mr. David Rose of New York City.

Our Dr. Stephen Jacobsen has brought the wearable type of artificial kidney to the point where we now have a promising proto- type. Jacobsen's wearable artificial kidney uses the single needle principle. A patient having an arteriovenous fistula will stick him- self once a day and will dialyze himself for one or two hours. Dur- ing the rest of the day he will be unencumbered by tubes or needles. This concept conforms with the newer trend to dialyze frequently for short periods of time rather than three times per week for six or ten hours. The wearable artificial kidney is small enough to fit into a large shoulder purse, and it can be applied wherever the wearer may happen to be. It is battery-powered and has a very low noise level (Fig. 3).

At this time, it appears likely that it will be possible to use cartridges holding 200 g charcoal with some aluminum dioxide (as is done by the Japanese) to remove the phosphates, and some resin, such as Kayexalate, may also be added to the cartridge to remove potassium. Dr. Dharnidharka indicated that one liter of ultrafil- trate removed per 24 hours would suffice to take care of water and electrolyte removal. As long as we do not have a specific urea ad- sorbent for this artificial kidney, conventional dialysis will be nec- essary from time to time to remove the urea. Normal persons form 20-40 g urea per 24 hours.

The Japanese, in the meantime, have obtained experience with a small type of artificial kidney for home dialysis which has only 30 l dialyzing fluid, but a large cartridge with 500 g charcoal. The blood urea nitrogen of the patient is allowed to go up to 140, but the Japanese claim that this does not impair the well-being of the pa- tient.

With work done in various places on oxystarches and aldehydes, and a new type of electrolysis, it is likely that in the near future, other and better ways will be found to remove urea.

Peritoneal Lavage. This is a method that competes with the artificial kidney and, we believe, will be particularly useful in the treatment of diabetics who do poorly on hemodialysis, for small children, and for patients who have run out of blood access sites. An international team comprised of Dr. Haapanen from Finland, Dr. Foux from Israel, and Dr. Houtchens, Messrs. Luntz, Nielsen and Kirkham from the U.S., are working on a peritoneal lavage machine that depends on reverse osmosis to produce a sterile,

inexpensive dialyzing fluid and will dispense it to the patient auto-
matically in the exact amount to give proper fluid balance (Fig. 4).
Reverse osmosis also removes undesirable substances such as excess calcium, excess iron, fluoride, etc. from the water. At this
time, however, we doubt that peritoneal lavage by reverse osmosis
will suffice for sterilization.

Single Needle Dialysis. Single needle dialysis, introduced by
Dr. Klaus Kopp in our laboratory three years ago, is gaining clinical acceptance. While our own patients use it successfully in home
dialysis, it is becoming obvious that it can be misused. Additional
work to explain the method to nonbelievers is now becoming useful
(Fig. 5).

EZS Kidney. Our EZS type of artificial kidney has as its claim
the fact that it saves the patient $1,500 per year when compared
with the use of a disposable kidney for each dialysis (Fig. 6).

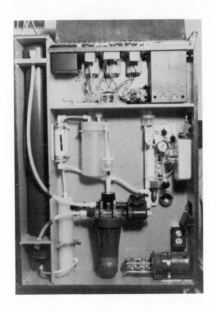

FIGURE 4. Dr. Houtchens' peritoneal dialysis machine using
reverse osmosis. It proved to be less simple than method proposed.

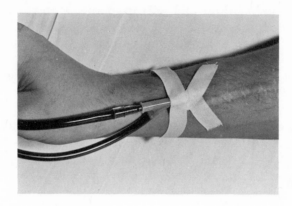

FIGURE 5. Single needle dialysis uses a Y connector. Blood goes in and out through a single needle when the tubes of the Y are alternatingly closed.

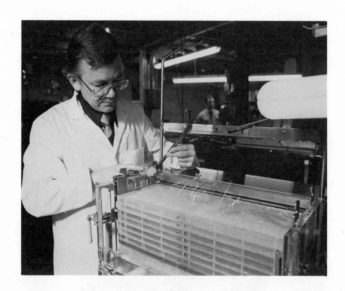

FIGURE 6. EZS Kidney shown with Mr. David Radford who built it. Presterilized wide cellophane, Cuprophane or Nephrophane tubing is placed between the plates of this dialyzer. It saves money because so little is thrown away after use.

Now that HR-1 has been signed into law, patients suffering from terminal kidney disease can qualify for federal help if they are covered by Social Security. We believe that it is mandatory that inexpensive means of dialysis be further accepted since otherwise, Congress may regret having brought help for our fellow citizens in terminal kidney disease. It has been estimated that in the U. S. we will have 40, 000 people on maintenance dialysis within a few years. If all of them have institutional dialysis rather than home dialysis, the difference being $20, 000 per patient per year, the total difference would be 800 million dollars per year. People will question whether or not it is justified to spend that much money for a small fraction of our population, even when they recognize that these people deserve help. Home dialysis, instead of institutional dialysis ($5, 000 vs $25, 000), and inexpensive dialysis vs expensive kidneys seem to offer the best answer.

Vacation Dialysis on Wheels. Anyone who knows that artificial kidney patients are bound to their machine three times per week will realize that it is difficult for these people to go on a vacation. To be dialyzed in another dialysis center is sometimes possible and sometimes prohibitively expensive. Mr. Albert Kolff wrote an illustrated brochure in which he explained the possibilities of vacation dialysis on wheels. On March 2, 1973, the Rotary Club of Murray, Utah, encouraged by Mr. and Mrs. Proctor, donated a beautiful trailer to the Division of Artificial Organs. An artificial kidney can be placed inside. The trailer is a modern one with bath, shower, flush toilet, built-in range, air conditioning, and heat. It sleeps six persons. It is available for patients on dialysis for a fee not higher than what is required to cover the expense (Fig. 7).

NAPHT. A local chapter of the National Association of Patients on Hemodialysis and Transplantation (NAPHT) was started with a dinner meeting on March 7, 1973 which the Division of Artificial Organs hosted. One hundred and eight people accepted the invitation. We believe that people sustained with artificial kidneys and people who have kidney transplants can help each other immensely with their problems. Dialysis centers throughout the country should help in getting local chapters started.*

---

*National Association of Patients on Hemodialysis and Transplantation, 505 Northern Blvd., Great Neck, N.Y. 11021, Mrs. Josephine Berman, President.

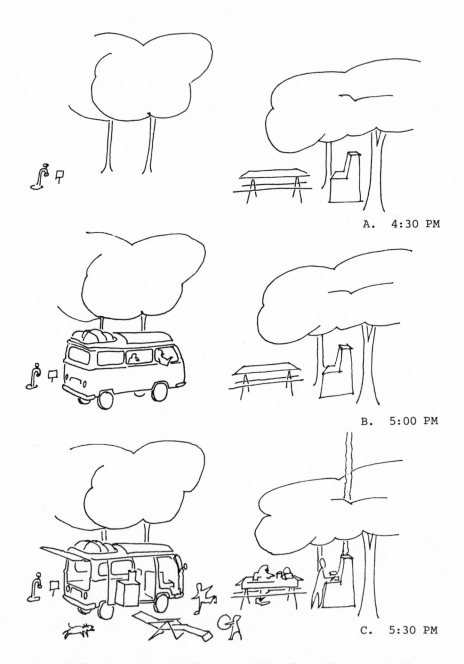

A.   4:30 PM

B.   5:00 PM

C.   5:30 PM

FIGURE 7. Vacation Dialysis on Wheels. Upon arrival at the camp site, the artificial kidney swings out of the VW bus.

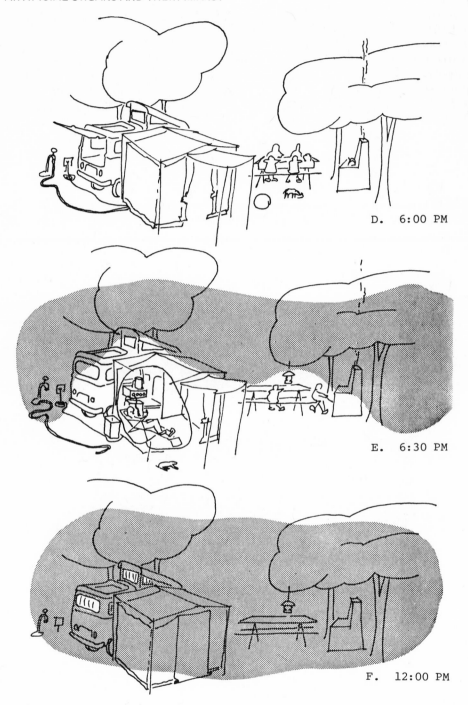

D.   6:00 PM

E.   6:30 PM

F.   12:00 PM

Dialysis in the tent. (By Albert Kolff, architect).

New Blood Vessels. Our Dr. Jay Volder has been successful in growing new blood vessels in sheep using the technique pioneered by Charles H. Sparks. Sparks inserts a Silastic rod covered with a double Dacron knit stocking into tissues of the animal or of the patient, and after six weeks, a tube is formed of host connective tissue having a Dacron skeleton. At that time the Silastic insert is pulled out. One end of such a tube is connected to an artery and the other to a vein. The tube can be punctured to obtain the necessary blood for patients on hemodialysis. Porous Teflon grafts (Gore-Tex) work equally well and have the advantage that they are immediately available for puncture (Fig. 8) [1]. For those thousands of kidney patients the world over who suffer from lack of blood vessels, infected shunts, or clotted arteriovenous fistulae, this is indeed very hopeful news.

THE ARTIFICIAL LIVER

Patients in coma due to liver disease have little chance of recovery, although some can now be saved with newer drugs and newer methods. Dr. David Hume and others have perfused the blood of these patients through the liver of baboons. Not only was temporary improvement observed, but some of these patients have

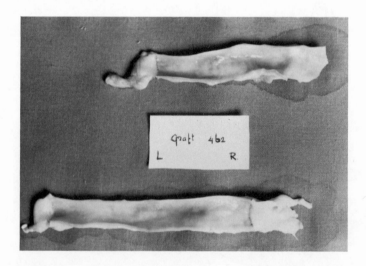

FIGURE 8. Dr. Jay Volder showed that arteriovenous grafts from porous material develop a beautiful intima and can be used for repeated puncturing (ASAIO 1974).

ultimately recovered. Liver transplantation, of which Dr. Starzel
in Denver is the main proponent, has been disappointing in its
clinical results. Many years ago, the Japanese tried to use an
emulsion of liver cells to exert their enzymatic action on the patient's blood, which was separated from these emulsions by cellophane membranes. Dr. N. Imaizumi, a Japanese surgeon who
worked with us for two years and who recently returned to Japan,
worked diligently on this problem while he was here. He was ad-
vised by Drs. James Freston, Frank Moody, Joseph Andrade and
W. J. Kolff. He cut fresh sheep liver into thin slices. There has
been an indication of activity of these cells when perfused with special Tyrode's solution, both for fresh slices and freeze-dried liver
material [2]. In the meantime, there is news that perfusion of
blood over (coated) charcoal may aid the removal of toxins from
the blood of patients otherwise dying in liver coma. Dr. E. Denti
from Italy recently joined our group to advance the program of the
artificial liver. He isolates the microsomes of liver cells for their
enzymatic activity.

THE ARTIFICIAL ARM

Artificial limbs constituted a field in which we wished to work
when I wrote up the initial program for the Institute for Biomedical
Engineering. We are extremely fortunate to have Dr. Steve
Jacobsen, who originally trained with us before receiving his Ph.D.
at M.I.T., working with us once more. To date, he has achieved
very important progress towards perfecting an artificial arm:

He has developed a very clever, light and powerful artificial
muscle which converts the rotary action of a small electric motor into linear motion.

He has developed better electrodes to pick up electrical
signals from muscles.

He has worked out mathematically a control system for movement of an artificial arm, when only myoelectric signals
from the shoulder muscles are available.

Dr. Jacobsen holds a position in the College of Engineering,
has an appointment in the Institute for Biomedical Engineering and,
via the Division of Artificial Organs, also has an appointment in
the Department of Surgery. We will combine his plans with the

facilities of our Microcircuit Laboratory, and I expect that a functional arm will be born which will compare favorably with anything
that is presently available. With the large number of young am-
putees from the Vietnam War, this seems to be a timely project
(Fig. 9).

COMPUTER GRAPHICS

Our Dr. Harvey Greenfield has opened an entirely new scientific field in biomedical engineering. He has introduced computer
graphics into medicine. The computer of the Advanced Computer
Center at the University of Utah in the College of Engineering
draws diagrams and objects on oscilloscopes. The drawings are
never touched by human hands, but are derived exclusively from
mathematical equations programmed into the computer. In previous years, he had demonstrated that areas of high turbulence in
the aorta coincide with those where atherosclerosis seems to begin.
He has now extended his studies to pulsatile flow and demonstrated,
in three-dimensional drawings (Fig. 10), that extremely high turbulence also occurs at the inflow and outflow openings of artificial
hearts (not properly shaped). The turbulence around a filling disc
valve is also clearly shown (Fig. 11). Dr. Greenfield and associates have demonstrated the stresses that occur in a ball made of
Silastic with photostress material subjected to actual pressure on
a ring.

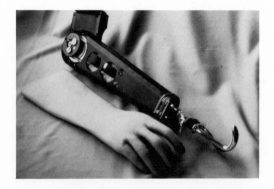

FIGURE 9. Artificial arm developed by Dr. Steve Jacobsen and
associates at the University of Utah. It has very light, powerful
muscles inside.

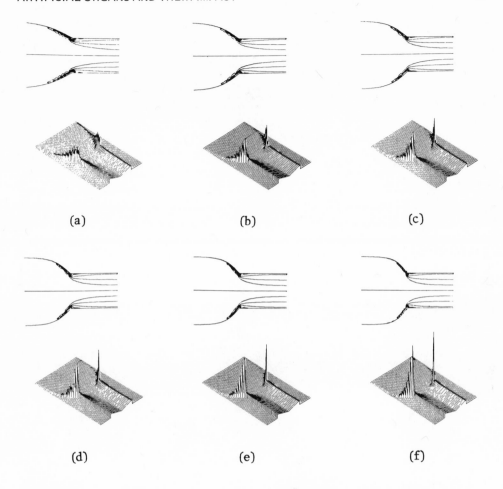

(a)   (b)   (c)

(d)   (e)   (f)

FIGURE 10.   Computer graphics by Harvey Greenfield and associates applied to artificial ventricle.   Time frames chosen from a
series of vorticity plots, showing systolic-diastolic motion of an
idealized, artificial ventricle.

     The equations were then fed into a computer which duplicated
the stress figures that had been found earlier.   We hope that this
new field opened for biomedical engineering by Dr. Greenfield can
be further developed, perhaps as a cooperative venture with the
Technion Institute in Haifa, Israel.

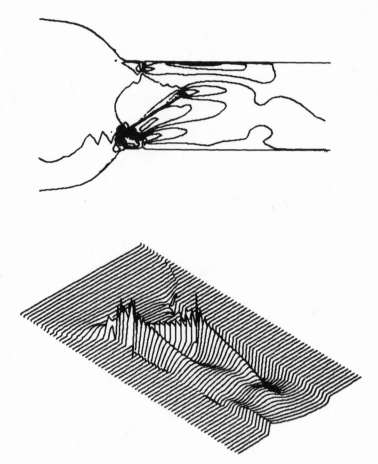

FIGURE 11. Turbulence around a filled disc valve, also drawn by computer graphics.

THE MICROCIRCUIT LABORATORY

The Institute for Biomedical Engineering, through the planning of our Mr. Dobelle, has obtained an entire experimental micro-circuit laboratory where production of complicated microcircuits can be carried out in their entirety. Microcircuits are immensely complex electrical circuits that are reproduced in several layers, all of which are superimposed on a small chip, the dimensions of which are often smaller than one-fourth of an inch squared (Fig. 12). To accomplish this, the original drawings, the size of a large win-dow, are reduced photographically 500 times. This is a 500 times

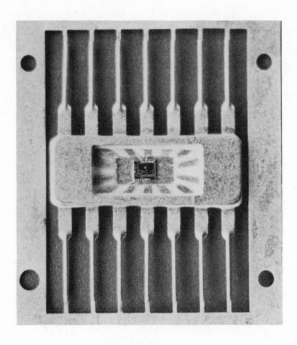

FIGURE 12. Microcircuit made by Dr. Robert Huber and associates at the University of Utah. Only the small square in the center
is the microcircuit (6,000 transistors, 6,000 diodes).

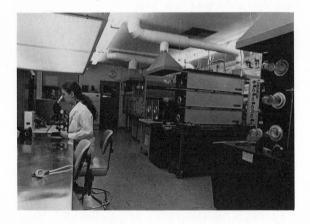

FIGURE 13. Microcircuit Laboratory. Some of the ovens are on
the right.

linear reduction which results in a 250,000 times area reduction. Our integrated microcircuit laboratory, with its photoengraving process, etc., is now in full operation (Fig. 13). This capability offers entirely new possibilities for the University of Utah Institute for Biomedical Engineering. Microcircuits are not at all or hardly ever used in medicine because the high volume, low unit profit industry which makes them cannot be bothered to make less than 50,000 items of one type.

Our Microcircuit Laboratory is presently financed by industry. It offers us the opportunity of introducing microcircuits into the biomedical field. The possible applications stagger the imagination. Microcircuits should be used in pacemakers (hardly done commercially, although 30,000 are placed into people every year) and in better electrodes to detect electrocardiograms or electro-myograms because the preamplifiers can then be built into the chip. An extremely able staff has been assembled in our Microcircuit Laboratory. Dr. Robert Huber is the Technical Director. There are physicists, engineers, a chemist, and a computer scientist on the staff. Each one has had industrial experience.

Without proper microcircuits, an artificial eye can never be made. It is now certain that an artificial ear can be approached. The House brothers and their co-workers in Los Angeles can obtain useful audible perception via a stimulating wire introduced through the foramen rotundum into the cochlea of some stone deaf individuals. To go back to the eye, I have seen the delight expressed by a totally blind person when his wires were stimulated with the computer setup by Mr. Mladejovsky and Mr. Dobelle.

In extensive stimulation of the brains of cats, a capacitor-coupled positive-negative waveform has been developed that, according to our Suzanne Stensaas, causes little or no detectable damage to the brain even on electron microscopy, i.e., examination. The first papers on our work on the artificial eye and the artificial ear have been published [3, 4, 5].

THE ARTIFICIAL EYE

Our traveling team of Dobelle, Mladejovsky, Dulmage and others has participated in the stimulation of the brains of patients who had the posterior part of their skulls open anyway since they required operations for brain tumors or other reasons. Since

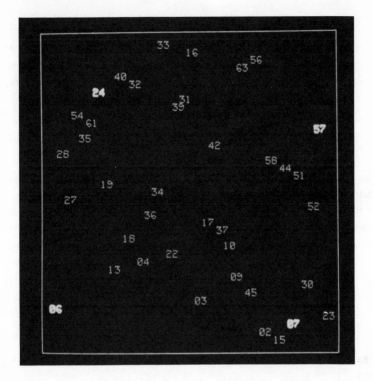

FIGURE 14. Phosphene map created by stimulation of the brain
of a blind volunteer. Each number indicates one electrode. When
the four points indicated in the corners were stimulated, he saw
four points that formed a square.

these operations are rare, particularly under local anesthesia,
our team traveled to 22 different neurosurgical clinics to accumulate an experience covering 34 patients. It became apparent that
one conscious patient could give so much more information than
the best trained monkey, that we ended up by donating our monkeys
to the zoo. Having confirmed earlier work by Penfield and Brindley
showing that stimulation of the occipital lobes of the brain can emu-
late "phosphenes" (the seeing of light points), we came to a point
where only blind volunteers could give us additional information.
Two longtime members of our blind advisory panel went with our
entire team to London, Ontario, Canada. Dr. John Girvin placed
an array of 64 electrodes on the mesial side of the occipital lobe
of each blind volunteer, and electrical stimulation started. One
volunteer, having been blind for 28 years, saw silvery white lights

upon stimulation of each of 45 electrodes. I asked him how it felt and he said, "When you have not seen anything for nearly 30 years, it is very pleasant to see something". He saw the silvery white spots floating in space, at arm's length and apparently all of them in one plane. The other volunteer, having lost both eyes in Vietnam seven years previously when a grenade exploded near his face, could see lights upon stimulation of 60 electrodes. A so-called phosphene map was constructed to determine the relative position of each phosphene in the visual field (Fig. 14). When four points were stimulated, he could see them, and without hesitation, told us they formed a square. We are aiming for a mobile prosthesis, something that will allow blind people to walk without bumping into things. Figure 15 shows the concept of the artificial eye. Two hundred thousand people are legally blind in the U. S. and less than _ ten percent can use Braille. Our artificial eye will not require training. The subject cannot help but see white dots when his brain is stimulated. However, for each individual patient, a computer analysis will be required to define the relationship between the electrodes of the array and the points they form in the visual field. We know how to do it.

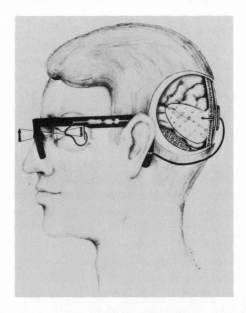

FIGURE 15. Diagram of concept of artificial eye. Television cameras in the glasses relate the message via microcomputers with radiowaves to the array of electrodes on the visual cortex of the brain.

PICKING UP SIGNALS FROM THE BRAIN

Picking up signals from the brain by application of microcircuit technology is another possibility. Thus, a man paralyzed
from the neck down might yield signals from his motor cortex,
enough to innervate his paralyzed limbs. The treatment of pain
by stimulation of certain parts of the brain or spinal cord, perhaps
even the changes of mood, are future possibilities. Temporary
stimulation would certainly be preferable to irreversible forms of
psychosurgery which are now widely criticized.

EXPLORATION OF CARDIAC ASSIST DEVICES AND
REVASCULARIZATION OF THE MYOCARDIUM

The intra-aortic balloon pump which we introduced in 1961 as
a cardiac assist device aimed at sustaining the circulation and for
relieving a failing heart is now the most popular and most used of
all assist devices, largely thanks to the persistence of Adrian and
Arthur Kantrowitz. More recently, Dr. Hans Zwart developed the
transarterial bypass which has been explored widely in our experimental laboratory, but has not yet gained clinical acceptance. With
the increased use of heart-lung machines to repair the coronary
circulation, there are a number of patients whose hearts are too
weak at the end of the operation to carry the circulation. Since
the chest is already open in these cases, a transapical form of
cardiac assist can be instituted within three minutes. A double
lumen catheter is introduced with a stylet through the apex of the
left ventricle. A longer inner cannula protrudes into the aorta,
and a wider outer cannula remains in the ventricle. The blood
flows out from the left ventricle and is pumped back into the aorta.
Thus, circulation can be sustained even when the heart is fibril-
lating (Fig. 16). We have recently reactivated this program and
hope to combine it with a new method for providing blood to a specific area of the myocardium that has an irreparably occluded coronary artery.

BLOOD TO ISCHEMIC MYOCARDIUM

Following the advice of our friend and yearly consultant,
Dr. S. Moulopoulos, we created an anastomosis between the mammary artery and the specific vein that drains the ischemic area of
the heart muscle. In experimental animals, we have records to

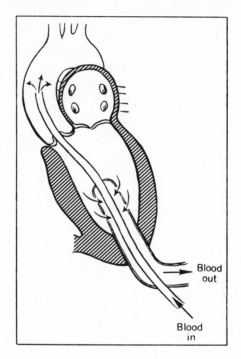

FIGURE 16. Diagram of transapical bypass. Remove the blood from the ailing ventricle and pump it back into the aorta.

show that indeed, oxygenated blood reaches the ischemic myocardium when it cannot get there via an occluded artery. The method is aimed at immediate vascularization following a severe heart attack to avert irrecoverable ischemic damage when it is impossible to create blood supply via the usual arterial route (Fig. 17). We believe this method and others presently under investigation in our laboratory may save the lives of 100,000 people per year in the U.S. alone.

THE ARTIFICIAL HEART [6]

Some 600,000 people die every year in the U.S. from the common coronary heart attack. Some 100,000 die from other heart diseases. Obviously there will never be enough human hearts for transplantation. Even if the problem of immune rejection can be overcome, the problems of procurement of human natural hearts remain insurmountable, whereas once we know how to make an artificial heart, we will be able to make as many as are needed.

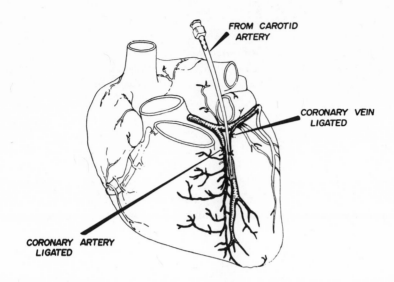

FIGURE 17. Diagram of heart with coronary vein perfused. When the coronary artery is tied off, ischemic necrosis of the myocardium is prevented when the blood reaches it through the vein that normally drains the area.

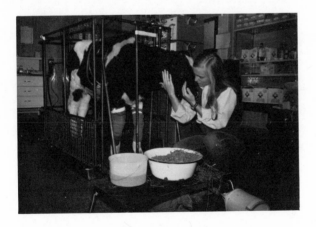

FIGURE 18. "Tony" on the 33rd day after removal of its natural heart and replacement by an artificial pump. This world record has now been improved by our calf, "Burke", surviving 45 days. (Principal Investigator: Dr. D. Olsen).

We recently succeeded in sustaining a calf for 45 days* with an artificial heart after its natural heart had been removed (Fig. 18). The calf was ambulatory, ate, drank, and had normal body functions. A series of animals surviving between a week and 36 days revealed that the following problems are not entirely solved, although great progress has been made as will be discussed in the following pages.

Disseminated Intravascular Coagulation (D.I.C.). Small clots initiated inside the artificial heart break loose, become lodged in other parts of the body and continue to develop there. They may use up the normal clotting factors, resulting in what is called consumptive coagulopathy which may lead to bleeding. During the last two years, this coagulopathy in our animals has been compensated and no longer leads to bleeding tendencies.

To overcome D.I.C., we used rough surfaces on the inside of our artificial hearts to prevent clots from dislodging. We have used Dacron fibrils, but since the Dacron fibrils did not adhere well to Silastic, we are in the process of converting to polyurethane substrates for the artificial heart. Indeed, it seems that D.I.C. is no longer a generalized problem in our recent experiments, although local clot formation remains a problem. We are now at the point where we can make our most successful artificial heart, the Jarvik Heart, of smooth polyurethanes. Indeed, the present world champion calf has a polyurethane heart with a smooth intima (Biomer**).

Respiratory Distress Syndrome (R.D.S). This is similar to the condition found in premature babies and in patients in severe shock from any cause where the lungs, for reasons not totally understood, lose a great deal of their capacity to oxygenate blood. If it is progressive, it may be fatal.

R.D.S. has lost much of its threat and danger in our recent experiments.

A Syndrome Comparable with Right Heart Failure. This was totally unexpected, but we have unequivocably shown, in many

---

*Editors' note added in proof: This calf survived for over 90 days, a new world's record.

**Ethicon, Inc., Somerville, N. J.

animals, that the venous pressure continues to increase, the blood volume increases, the liver becomes large and congested, and fluid may accumulate in the abdomen. It is our belief at this time that this is caused by (1) improper fit of the artificial heart that compresses the veins; (2) improper action of the atria, either the remnants of the natural atria or the artificial atria; (3) regurgitation and other malfunctions of the atrioventricular valve, and (4) the fact that our artificial hearts which respond to Starling's Law should respond with a steeper curve than they presently do.

To avoid the syndrome of right heart failure, the most important factor seems to be to make a heart with adequate output that fits inside the chest without compressing the veins. Our Robert Jarvik developed an artificial heart of a new design on which he worked for one and a half years (Fig. 19). It was implanted for the first time on March 1, 1973. The ventrodorsal dimensions of this artificial heart are considerably smaller than those of the previously used Kwan-Gett heart. At the time of writing, the calves

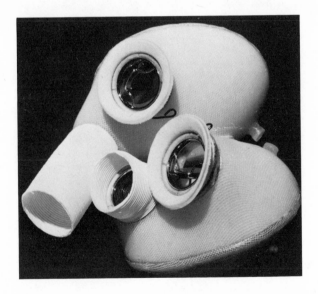

FIGURE 19. Jarvik Heart. The essential improvement made by Dr. Jarvik is the small ventrodorsal dimension of this heart. It avoids compression of the venous structures (veins) dorsal to the heart.

with this artificial heart have lower venous pressures than other calves ever had, and this remains so unless local thrombus formation interferes with valve function.

Our Dr. Jeffrey Peters and Mr. Tom Kessler have produced artificial hearts that have compliant atria, the outer wall of which is rigid while the inner wall is compliant, the space in between being vented to the atmosphere. These hearts seem to improve cardiac output greatly and may prevent sucking in the wall of the vena cava which we previously saw when a slightly subatmospheric pressure was used to fill the artificial ventricles.

To study the function of the artificial heart accurately, our former associate and present consultant, Dr. Frank Donovan, developed a mock circulation which, without any instrumentation on the artificial heart itself, accurately determines stroke volume, cardiac output, etc.

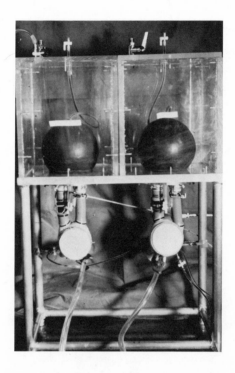

FIGURE 20. Dr. Peters' mock circulation. Blood damage done by two ventricles can be compared in identical systems.

Hemolytic Icterus. This is a jaundice which originates on the basis of breakdown of red blood cells. It is amazing because this breakdown is so small that it cannot be detected from the color of the blood plasma. Yet, we believe we have proven beyond doubt that the icterus is hemolytic.

Dr. Jeffrey Peters, together with several students, has tested the hemolytic damage of artificial hearts in a special system which uses fresh cow blood and, in itself, is not hemolytic (Fig. 20). It was clear that rough surfaces such as velour which had been used earlier produce more hemolysis than fine fibril surfaces, and these cause more hemolysis than smooth surfaces. It is most encouraging that the calf, "Burke", presently living 45 days after implantation of the artificial heart, has no trace of hemolytic icterus. It has not needed any blood transfusions after the first postoperative day. Its artificial heart has an intima of smooth polyurethane (Biomer).

ARTIFICIAL HEART DRIVEN BY ATOMIC ENERGY*

Our Mr. Lee Smith and Dr. Gary Sandquist are in charge of our program to produce an artificial heart driven by atomic energy. Most of our other artificial hearts are driven by power sources outside the body; this necessitated six-foot-long tubes for the driving air, coming from the driving system outside the chest. Of course, this has disadvantages, but we felt that much could be learned with this method. Moreover, we felt that there are people who would prefer to live and walk around with a moveable cart, rather than die.

The artificial heart driven by atomic energy can be totally contained within the body. The power is derived from plutonium 238. It gives off very little hard radiation and is contained in a steel capsule smaller than a Grade C egg. This capsule produces 33 watts; the artificial heart itself uses about six watts. Prototypes of this artificial heart driven by an electric motor have been implanted in animals. One calf lived for 69 hours and several were able to stand up. The soft shell design which we developed a few

---

*This is a collaborative program with Westinghouse, North American Phillips, and is supervised and financed by the Atomic Energy Commission.

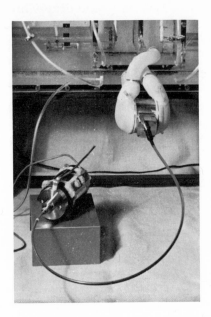

FIGURE 21. Prototype AEC heart with long drive shaft while tested in a mock circulation. Only six watts are required to drive this heart, measured at the motor end of the shaft.

years ago is used for the ventricles and makes the artificial heart respond to venous pressure (Starling's Law) without the need for electronic controls (Fig. 21).

HOW OUR INSTITUTE GROWS AND DEVELOPS

Great activity is occurring in all the fields in which the Institute for Biomedical Engineering is active. Those in the field of instrumentation, headed by Dr. Curtis Johnson, have not even been discussed here. Our general policies remain the same:

1. Try to obtain funding from private sources so that we can prove the feasibility of a given project, then try to fund it further from Government sources or from industry. "Seed" money is extremely important.

2. Stress the quality of our scientific personnel, not buildings. Provide the personnel with adequate equipment, but not

too much equipment. When we attract strong people, which we have done, they become self-sufficient, develop their own programs, and attract other strong people.

3. Encourage the members of our staff to engage in teaching, and assist them in obtaining academic appointments in their original disciplines. This will attract students who will become our future staff members and build a liaison with academic departments of the University which will make the Institute for Biomedical Engineering continuously viable in future years.

4. Since we are now well on our way to accomplishing what we started to do in 1967 when I joined the University of Utah, the time approaches to look for buildings based on the existing staff and programs, with space for future expansion in areas that are now clearly predictable. Indeed, the Legislature of the State of Utah has provided $664,000 which will be used for a building for experimental surgery in the study of the artificial heart. Additional buildings will have to be constructed as the funding becomes available.

REFERENCES

1.   Volder, J.G.R., Trans. Amer. Soc. Artif. Intern. Organs, 19, 38 (1973).

2.   Imaizumi, N., Kralios, N., Walker, J., Andrade, J. D., Freston, J. W., and Kolff, W. J., Abstracts, Annual Meeting of the American Society for Artificial Internal Organs, Chicago, Ill., April 3-5, 1974.

3.   Dobelle, W. H., Mladejovsky, M. G., Stensaas, S. S., and Smith, J. B., Ann. Otol. Rhinol. Laryngol., 82, 445 (1973).

4.   Dobelle, W. H., et al., Bringing Sight to the Blind, Electronics, January, 1974.

5.   Dobelle, W. H., Mladejovsky, M. G., and Girvin, J. P., Science, 183, 440 (1974).

6.   Kolff, W. J., Review of Literature, in Artificial Heart,
     Cardiac Assist Devices and Artificial Kidney, Harvey Papers -
     Technion in Haifa, Israel (in press).

BIOMEDICAL POLYMERS - AN INTRODUCTION

Donald J. Lyman

Department of Materials Science and Engineering
Department of Surgery (Division of Artificial Organs)
University of Utah, Salt Lake City, Utah

During this last decade we have seen not only a large increase in the number of polymers being examined for biomedical uses, but more significantly, a great change in how these materials were characterized. Luckily, we no longer see papers in which, for example, the author simply said, "a plastic was implanted"; and we are seeing less data simply being reported as gross observations only.

Much of this has occurred because of the recognition that this area of research is no longer the sole domain of the surgeon, but is truly interdisciplinary, requiring the blending of a number of talents. As a result, we are beginning to learn much more about the events that occur, at the molecular level, as we interface the polymer with the living system, events that affect the fate of the implant and the life of the patient. From these many in vitro and in vivo studies, we have set up questions that must be considered in any implant research experiment.

(1) Is the polymer pure? Almost all commercial polymers contain additives of various types including residual catalysts and solvents. While polymers prepared in the laboratory are often free from these impurities, features such as molecular weight distribution and abnormal linkages in the polymer structure must be considered. All of these can alter the performance of a given polymer.

(2) <u>Does the polymer have the necessary chemical, physical,</u>
<u>and mechanical properties for its proposed function</u>? Most im-
plant studies proceed rather empirically in matching polymer to
design and function. As a result, polymers are often forced into
situations where they should not be used. This problem will largely
disappear as the polymer scientist interacts more fully with the device maker and as more information concerning the interaction
between the polymer and the living system becomes available.

(3) <u>Can the polymer be fabricated into the desired implant</u>
<u>without a change in its properties</u>? The recent studies on surface
properties of polymers have shown how easily the surface can be
chemically altered (oxidized) or contaminated (by oils, mold release agents, etc.) by the fabrication technique. Also, some polymers give different results depending on whether the surface was
formed on the mold or the air side. We have also shown the adverse effect of residual solvents, especially N, N-dimethyl form-
amide, on blood reactions. In addition, changes in polymer crystallinity, domain structure of block copolymers, or the creation of
unusual stresses can occur in fabrication.

(4) <u>Can we sterilize the polymer without adversely affecting</u>
<u>its properties</u>? Polymers readily absorb many chemicals used in
sterilization procedures, and their surface properties are often
adversely changed unless the sterilant is fully removed. As a result, steam sterilization is the best method of sterilizing polymer
implants, if the heat distortion temperature of the material is not
below autoclave temperature. Many hospital steam systems contain additives which can absorb onto the polymer, thus compromis-
ing their function; therefore, polymer implants should be suitably
packaged or the autoclave should have its own water source for
generating steam.

However, cleanness of surface and sterility must be our goal
if we are to avoid biological problems on implantation.

(5) <u>Is the polymer adversely affected by the biological envi-</u>
<u>ronment</u>? The polymer properties must not change critically dur-
ing the time span of the implant. This can put severe restrictions
on long-term implant devices. While a polymer can be screened
for problems such as hydrolytic and oxidative degradation, and
lipid absorption, actual implantation is necessary to evaluate problems such as calcification and fibrous ingrowth, and to determine if
the implant conditions accelerate the anticipated degradation rates.

In addition to the factors outlined above, we must also consider how the polymer affects the living system. For example:

(6) <u>Does the polymer induce thrombus formation or adversely alter any of the blood constituents</u>? This is a particularly difficult area of study since both the polymer surface and blood flow conditions can influence the overall results. The use of computer graphics techniques in hemodynamics should allow the coupling of engineering design of implants to known effects of flowing blood with polymer surfaces.

(7) <u>Does the polymer induce any foreign body, inflammatory, encapsulation, or cell change response to the surrounding tissue?</u>

(8) <u>Does the polymer cause any antileukotactic response?</u>

(9) <u>Does the polymer induce any tumor formation</u>?

Studies on the above three questions would appear to profit from more detailed use of cell culture techniques and quantitation of the effects of implants on tissue.

Since the body has its own protection mechanism, all of these responses of the living system to the polymer will be dependent on factors such as the quantity of polymer in the implant, the site of implantation, the rate of degradation product formation, etc.

Two additional questions must also be considered. They are:

(10) <u>Does the implant have the proper design?</u>

(11) <u>Is the implantation procedure (and in some cases the post-operative care) proper to insure the best possible results?</u>

The best polymer can be compromised in its function by both the device designer or the implanting surgeon. My group has tried to avoid these problems by proper coupling of the basic polymer studies, device design and fabrication, and surgical approaches. This is done by requiring all of our group, scientist, engineer, or surgeon to essentially do a short "internship" in all sectors of the implant program and then establish the right team for a particular implant development.

During the remainder of this symposium, we will be returning again and again to the questions posed above as we look at a variety of polymers and implant devices.

REFERENCE

Lyman, D. J. and Seare, W. J., Jr., Ann. Rev. Mater. Sci. 4, 415 (1974).

HYDROGELS - A BROAD CLASS OF BIOMATERIALS

Allan S. Hoffman

Center for Bioengineering, University of Washington
Seattle, Washington 98195

INTRODUCTION

The term "hydrogel" refers to a broad class of polymeric
materials which are swollen extensively in water (30-90%) but
which do not dissolve in water. They have been used in a wide
variety and growing number of biomedical applications since they
often exhibit good biocompatibility. They may be applied in bulk
forms which vary from clear solids to opaque sponges; sometimes
these forms are reinforced by woven fabrics since the highly water-
swollen gels are mechanically weak. For this same reason, they
are also useful as coatings, especially when the biomedical application involves the contact of a preformed device or implant with
body fluids. Table I summarizes a number of applications of hydrogels which have been mentioned in the literature (see references
also).

It can be seen that some of the applications listed in Table I
require biological action as well as biocompatibility. Often this is
achieved by entrapping or immobilizing the active agent via chemical bonding, on or within the hydrogel. A summary of such active
agents is presented in Table II.

This paper summarizes the synthesis, composition, imbibed
water characterization, biological interactions and applications of
hydrogels. An extensive bibliography is presented at the end.

TABLE I

HYDROGELS MAY BE USED IN CONTACT WITH THE BODY
AS TISSUE AND BLOOD COMPATIBLE

<u>COATINGS</u>   OR   <u>"HOMOGENEOUS" MATERIALS</u>

Sutures   Contact lenses
Catheters   Artificial corneas
IUDs   Estrus-inducer
Blood detoxicant   Breast or other soft tissue
Sensors (electrodes)   substitutes
                                 Burn dressings
                                 Bone ingrowth sponge
                                 Dentures
                                 Ear drum plug

Therapeutic implant, device
Parts or the whole of artificial
   organs, vessels

TABLE II

HYDROGELS SOMETIMES MAY CONTAIN ENTRAPPED OR
IMMOBILIZED ACTIVE INGREDIENTS AS:

Antibiotics
Anticoagulants
Anticancer drugs
Antibodies
Drug antagonists
Enzymes
Contraceptives
Estrus-inducer
Antibacterial agents

SYNTHESIS AND COMPOSITION

As noted above, the term "hydrogel" refers to a wide variety of polymeric compositions. These materials may be synthesized from monomers or monomers mixed with polymers, or they may also be obtained by chemical modification of existing polymers.

Concerning the use of monomers, there are four basic classes of vinyl-type monomers which may be employed: neutral, acidic or anionic, basic or cationic, and crosslinker. Most of the monomers are hydrophilic, although one way to reduce water swelling, and thereby enhance mechanical strength, is by copolymerization of such monomers with hydrophobic monomers. Table III lists most of the vinyl-type monomers mentioned in the hydrogel literature.

Often a hydrogel may be synthesized or made into a useful form by physical or chemical conversion of existing polymers. A wide variety of possibilities exists for this route to hydrogels and Table IV summarizes a number of them. Note that in some cases the extent of chemical conversion will affect the water content of the swollen hydrogel. Since increase in water content leads to decrease in mechanical strength, optimization of these two opposing factors can be achieved.

When it is desired to coat a particular biomedical device or implant with a hydrogel, a number of different techniques based on the chemistry suggested in Tables III and IV may be used. These techniques are summarized in Table V.

CHARACTERIZATION OF THE IMBIBED WATER

In theory, hydrogels are attractive as biomaterials because they are similar to the body's own highly hydrated composition. Thus, if the interface of a foreign object does not appear foreign to the biomolecules and cells in the vicinity, then they should not be attracted to the interface. If they were to be strongly attracted to and strongly adherent at the interface of a foreign material, then it is entirely possible that they would be structurally distorted or biologically denatured by such strong interactions. Of course, some adherence of molecules and cells may be desirable in certain situations, as in the growth of endothelial cells over the inside surface of a synthetic vascular graft. Another biomedical advantage

TABLE III

MONOMERS USED IN HYDROGELS

NEUTRAL

HYDROXYMETHYL METHACRYLATE $\quad CH_2=C(CH_3)(CO_2C_2H_4OH)$

GLYCERYL METHACRYLATE $\quad CH_2=C(CH_3)(CO_2CH_2CH(OH)-CH_2OH)$

PROPYLENEGLYCOL METHACRYLATE $\quad CH_2=C(CH_3)(CO_2CH_2CH(OH)-CH_3)$

2,4 PENTADIENE-1-OL $\quad CH_2=CH-CH=CH-CH_2OH$

ACRYLAMIDE DERIVATIVES $\quad CH_2=C(R)-CO-N(R')(R'')$

$(R=-H,-CH_3)$
$(R,R''=-H,-CH_3-C_2H_5,-CH_2CHOHCH_3)$

N-VINYL PYRROLIDONE $\quad CH_2=CH-N$ (pyrrolidone ring)

ACRYLICS $\quad CH_2=C(R)(CO_2R')$

$(R=-H,-CH_3)$
$(R'=-CH_3,-C_4H_9)$

ACIDIC OR ANIONIC

ACRYLIC ACID, DERIVATIVES $\quad CH_2=C(R)-CO_2H$

$(R=-H,-CH_3)$

CROTONIC ACID $\quad CH_3-C=CH-CO_2H$ (with VAc)

SODIUM STYRENE SULFONATE $\quad CH_2=CH-\langle\text{ring}\rangle-SO_3^{\ominus} \; Na^{\oplus}$

BASIC OR CATIONIC

AMINOETHYL METHACRYLATE, DERIVATIVES $\quad CH_2=C(R)-CO_2-C_2H_4N-R'(R'')$

$(R,R',R''=-H,-CH_3,-C_4H_9)$

PYRIDENE $\quad CH_2=CH-\langle\text{pyridine ring}\rangle$

CROSSLINKERS

ETHYLENEGLYCOL DIMETHACRYLATE DERIVATIVES $\quad CH_2=C(R)-CO-O-(CH_2CH_2O)_x-CO-C(R)=CH_2$

METHYLENE-BIS-ACRYLAMIDE $\quad CH_2=CH-CO-NH-CH_2-NH-CO-CH=CH_2$

TABLE IV

CONVERTED POLYMERS USED AS HYDROGELS

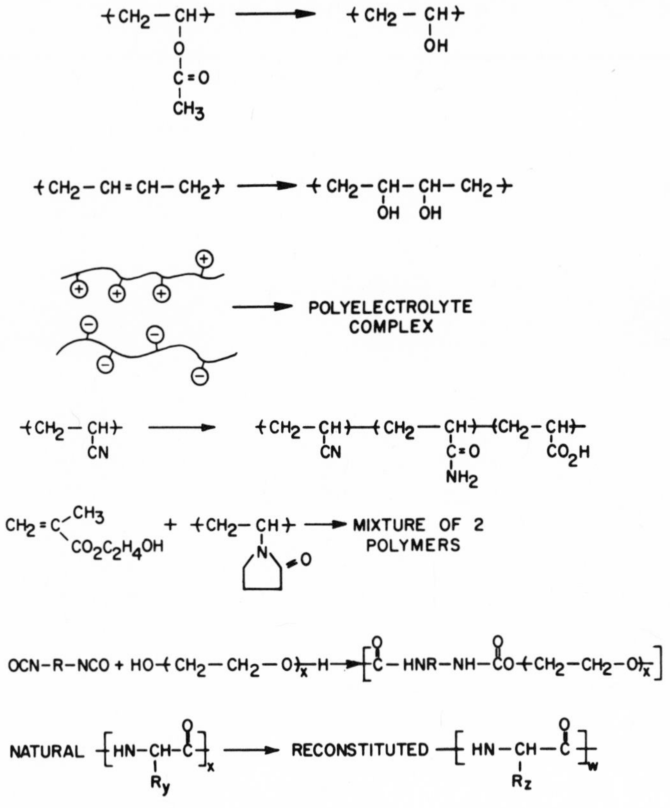

$$+CH_2-CH+ \underset{\substack{O \\ | \\ C=O \\ | \\ CH_3}}{} \longrightarrow +CH_2-\underset{\substack{| \\ OH}}{CH}+$$

$$+CH_2-CH=CH-CH_2+ \longrightarrow +CH_2-\underset{\substack{| \\ OH}}{CH}-\underset{\substack{| \\ OH}}{CH}-CH_2+$$

⟶ POLYELECTROLYTE COMPLEX

$$+CH_2-\underset{\substack{| \\ CN}}{CH}+ \longrightarrow +CH_2-\underset{\substack{| \\ CN}}{CH}+ +CH_2-\underset{\substack{| \\ C=O \\ | \\ NH_2}}{CH}+ +CH_2-\underset{\substack{| \\ CO_2H}}{CH}+$$

$$CH_2=C\underset{CO_2C_2H_4OH}{\overset{CH_3}{\diagdown}} + +CH_2-CH+ \longrightarrow \text{MIXTURE OF 2 POLYMERS}$$

$$OCN-R-NCO + HO+CH_2-CH_2-O)_x H \longrightarrow \left[\overset{O}{\overset{\|}{C}}-HNR-NH-\overset{O}{\overset{\|}{C}}O+CH_2-CH_2-O)_x \right]$$

$$\text{NATURAL} \left[HN-\underset{\substack{| \\ R_y}}{CH}-\overset{O}{\overset{\|}{C}} \right]_x \longrightarrow \text{RECONSTITUTED} \left[HN-\underset{\substack{| \\ R_z}}{CH}-\overset{O}{\overset{\|}{C}} \right]_w$$

TABLE V

HYDROGEL COATING TECHNIQUES

1. Dip-coat in prepolymer + solvent

2. Dip in monomer(s) ($\pm$ solvent, polymer) then
    polymerize using catalyst $\pm$ heat

3. Preactivate surface ("active vapor", ionizing
    radiation in air) then contact with monomers
    $\pm$ heat to polymerize

4. Irradiate with ionizing radiation while in con-
    tact with vapor or liquid solution of mono-
    mer(s)

of hydrogels may be related to their high permeabilities to water
and small ions or molecules.

Although the gross water contents of swollen hydrogels are
most easily measured and most often reported, the biological interaction at the hydrogel biological fluid interface may well be
directed by the organization of the water in the hydrogel. Concerning this point, hydrogel water may be (a) polarized around charged
ionic groups, (b) oriented around hydrogen bonding groups or other
dipoles, (c) structured around hydrophobic groups or (d) imbibed
in large pores as normal bulk water.

Attempts have been made to separate the total gel water content into some of these categories using NMR techniques [26, 28].
By use of NMR, the gel water content was divided into bulk water
(category d), bound water (categories a, b) and the remaining
water, termed interface water (category c). Results for a poly-
hydroxyethyl methacrylate (polyHEMA) gel suggest that a large
fraction (e.g. >50%) of the total gel water is imbibed as normal
bulk water, while smaller but significant fractions (e.g. perhaps
each 15-25%) exist as bound water (polarized or oriented around
ions, H-bonds, dipoles) and interface water (structured around
hydrophobic groups).

These results are only preliminary indications; furthermore, the effects of water organization on biological interactions remain to be elucidated. It should also be noted that the organization and content of absorbed gel water will vary significantly with hydrogel composition, probably most often in expected directions.

BIOLOGICAL INTERACTIONS

There is an extensive literature on the interaction of biomolecules, cells, tissue, and blood with hydrogels (see references).

Although it can be hazardous to make too many generalizations from these studies, there are, nonetheless, a few points which may be noted:

1) In the absence of specific interactions such as those due to acidic or basic ionic sites, hydrogels appear to adsorb proteins and adhere cells more gently than low water content foreign interfaces, as evidenced by the greater ease of desorption of adsorbed proteins and cells from poly-HEMA hydrogels grafted onto silicone rubber or polyurethane surfaces vs the original polymer surfaces [32, 33]. These phenomena may be due to the release of greater quantities of structured water (category c above) from the low water content, hydrophobic interfaces vs the hydrated, hydrogel interfaces when proteins or cells contact these interfaces. Subsequent desorption of such species would then be more difficult from the hydrophobic interfaces due to the need to break the hydrophobic bonding between the biological species and the foreign polymer, and readsorb and restructure water molecules at the interface. This is thermodynamically unfavorable [31].

2) Soft, collagenous tissue ingrowth increases as pore size increases in porous, opaque polyHEMA hydrogel sponges [34, 37]. There may be a change in the ingrowth behavior above 50-60% water content when ingrowth of blood capillaries is facilitated [39, 40].

3) Control of the composition and porosity of the hydrogel may encourage or discourage deposition of hard, calcified tissue within the gel pores [38, 40].

4) Blood compatibility of several hydrogel materials appears to be good, based on vena cava ring tests [43, 51, 53]. Embolus formation from some of these can occur, however [52], although this is probably typical of many foreign surfaces in contact with blood.

CONCLUDING REMARKS

Many different hydrogels appear to display good biocompatibility by a variety of tests. However, it is very important to identify and interrelate the hydrogel purity and composition, its water content and organization, the particular biological test used to evaluate the biocompatibility, and the ultimate biomedical application being considered on the basis of the test results. Much remains to be learned in all of these areas.

REFERENCES

General Articles on Biomedical Applications

1.   Wichterle, O. and Lim, D., Nature 165, 117 (1960).

2.   Levowitz, B. S., LaGuerre, J. N., Calem, W. S., Gould, F. E., Scherrer, J., and Schoenfeld, H., Trans. Amer. Soc. Artif. Intern. Organs, 14, 82 (1968).

3.   Bruck, S. D., J. Biomed. Mater. Res., 7, 387 (1973).

Contact Lens and Other Optical Applications

4.   Refojo, M. F., J. Biomed. Mater. Res., 3, 333 (1969).

5.   Laizier, J. and Wajs, G., in Proceedings on the Utilization of Large Radiation Sources and Accelerators in Industrial Processing, Munich, August 18-22, 1969, International Atomic Energy Agency, Vienna, 1970, p. 205.

6.   Refojo, M. F., J. Biomed. Mater. Res., 5, 113 (1971).

7.   Refojo, M. F., Surv. Ophthalmol., 16, 233 (1972).

8.   Holly, F. J. and Refojo, M. F., J. Amer. Optom. Assoc.
      43(11), 1 (1972).

9.   Refojo, M. F., in The Preocular Tear Film and Dry Eye
      Syndromes, F. J. Holly and M. A. Lemp, Eds., Int.
      Ophthal. Clin., 13(1), 1 (1973).

Applications Involving Delivery of Active Agents

10.   Tollar, M., Stol, M, and Kliment, K., J. Biomed. Mater.
      Res., 3, 305 (1969).

11.   Majkus, V., Horakova, Z., Vymola, F., and Stol, M., ibid.,
      3, 443 (1969).

12.   Abrahams, R. A. and Ronel, S. H., presented at the 8th
      Annual Meeting of the Association for the Advancement of
      Medical Instrumentation, Washington, D.C., March 21-24,
      1973.

13.   Nathan, P., et al., Crit. Rev. Clin. Lab. Sci., 4, 61 (1973).

14.   Drobnik, J., Spacek, P., and Wichterle, O., J. Biomed.
      Mater. Res., 8, 45 (1974).

15.   Molday, R. S., Dreyer, W. J., Rembaum, A., and Yen,
      S.P.S., Nature, 249, 81 (1974).

Synthesis and Characterization of Structure, Composition, Water
Content and Organization

16.   Yasuda, H. and Refojo, M. F., J. Polym. Sci., 2, 5093
      (1964).

17.   Refojo, M. F. and Yasuda, H., J. Appl. Polym. Sci., 9,
      2425 (1965).

18.   Jadwin, T. A., Hoffman, A. S., and Vieth, W. R., ibid.,
      14, 1339 (1970).

19.   Ratner, B. D. and Miller, I. F., J. Polym. Sci. Pt. A-1,
      10, 2425 (1972).

20. Refojo, M. F., An. Quim., **68**, 697 (1972).

21. Hoffman, A. S. and Kraft, W. G., Amer. Chem. Soc., Div. Polym. Chem., Prepr., **13**, 723 (1972).

22. Lee, H. B., Shim, H. S., and Andrade, J. D., ibid., **13**, 729 (1972).

23. Hoffman, A. S. and Harris, C., ibid., **13**, 740 (1972).

24. Ratner, B. D. and Hoffman, A. S., Amer. Chem. Soc., Div. Org. Coat. Plast. Chem., Prepr., **33**, 286 (1973).

25. Andrade, J. D., Lee, H. B., Jhon, M. S., Kim, S. W., and Hibbs, J. B., Jr., Trans. Amer. Soc. Artif. Intern. Organs, **19**, 1 (1973).

26. Jhon, M. S. and Andrade, J. D., J. Biomed. Mater. Res. **7**, 509 (1973).

27. Bray, J. C. and Merrill, E. W., J. Appl. Polym. Sci., **17**, 3779 (1973).

28. Lee, H. B., Andrade, J. D., and Jhon, M. S., Amer. Chem. Soc., Div. Polym. Chem., Prepr., **15**, 706 (1974).

29. Meaburn, G. M., et al., Abstracts of the 5th International Congress of the Radiation Research Society, Seattle, Wash., July 14-21, 1974, p. 200.

30. Ratner, B. D. and Hoffman, A. S., J. Appl. Polym. Sci., **18**, 3183 (1974).

In Vitro Interactions with Proteins, Cells

31. Hoffman, A. S., J. Biomed. Mater. Res., 1974 (in press).

32. Horbett, T. A. and Hoffman, A. S., in Proteins on or as Substrates, Advances in Chemistry Series, American Chemical Society, Washington, D.C., 1974-75 (in press).

33. Ratner, B. D., et al., submitted for publication in Biomater., Med. Devices, Artif. Organs, 1974.

Interactions with Tissue

34.   Barvic, M., Kliment, K., and Zavadil, M., J. Biomed.
      Mater. Res., 1, 313 (1967).

35.   Kocvara, S., Kliment, C., Kubat, L., Stol, M., Ott, Z.,
      and Dvorak, J., ibid., 1, 325 (1967).

36.   Hubacek, J., Kliment, K., Dusek, J., and Hubacek, Jar,
      ibid., 1, 387 (1967).

37.   Chvapil, M., Holusa, R., Kliment, K., and Stol, M., ibid.,
      3, 315 (1969).

38.   Winter, G. D. and Simpson, B. J., Nature, 223, 88 (1969).

39.   Sprincl, L., Kopecek, J., and Lim, D., J. Biomed. Mater.
      Res., 5, 447 (1971).

40.   Sprincl, L., Vacik, J., and Kopecek, J., ibid., 7, 123
      (1973).

41.   Scott, H., Kronick, P. L., May, R. C., Davis, R. H.,
      and Balin, H., Biomater., Med. Devices, Artif. Organs, 1,
      681 (1973).

Interactions with Blood

42.   Singh, M. P., Biomed. Eng., 4, 68 (1968).

43.   Gott, V. L. and Baier, R. E., Report on Contract
      PH-43-68-84, NHLI, NIH, Bethesda, Md., U. S. Nat. Tech.
      Inform. Serv., PB Rept. No. 197,622, 1970.

44.   Merrill, E. W., Salzman, E. W., Wong, P.S.L., Ashford,
      T. P., Brown, A. H., and Austen, W. G., J. Appl. Physiol.,
      29, 723 (1970).

45.   Halpern, B. D., et al., Annual Reports on Contract
      PH-43-66-1124, NHLI, NIH, Bethesda, Md., U. S. Nat.
      Tech. Inform. Serv., PB Rept. Nos. 200,987, 1971;
      212,724, 1972; 215,886, 1973; 230,310, 1974.

46. Marshall, D. W., Annual Report on Contract PH-43-66-1129, NHLI, NIH, Bethesda, Md., PB Rept. No. 198,403, 1971.

47. Scott, H., et al., Annual Report on Contract NIH-NHLI-71-2017, NHLI, NIH, Bethesda, Md., PB Rept. Nos. 206,499, 1971; 221,846, 1973; 230,308, 1974.

48. Andrade, J. D., Kunitomo, K., Van Wegenen, R., Kastigir, B., Gough, D., and Kolff, W. J., Trans. Amer. Soc. Artif. Intern. Organs, 17, 222 (1971).

49. Hoffman, A. S., Schmer, G., Harris, C., and Kraft, W. G., ibid., 18, 10 (1972).

50. Kearney, J. J., et al., Amer. Chem. Soc., Div. Org. Coat. Plast. Chem., Prepr., 33, 286 (1973).

51. Kwiatkowski, G. T., et al., Annual Report on Contract NIH-71-2067-2, 1973, NHLI, NIH, Bethesda, Md.

52. Kusserow, B., et al., Annual Report on Contract PH-43-68-1427-2, 1971, NHLI, NIH, Bethesda, Md.

53. Ratner, B. D., et al., Biomater., Med. Devices, Artif. Organs, 1975 (in press).

NECESSARY CONSIDERATIONS FOR SELECTING A POLYMERIC MATERIAL FOR IMPLANTATION WITH EMPHASIS ON POLYURETHANES

Garth L. Wilkes

Polymer Materials Program, Department of Chemical Engineering, Princeton University, Princeton, New Jersey 08540

I. INTRODUCTION

It is best to begin this paper by stating that its content is intended primarily for those in the medical or medically related professions and for those who have a general need to understand or be aware of design problems concerned with polymeric implant materials. The word "design" is meant to be broad in meaning for this context in that the actual design considerations should begin with the chemistry used in producing the individual polymer chains and extend through the clinical testing of the fabricated device or implant.

To cover all of these considerations in complete detail would be difficult if not impossible for a single author. This is obvious from the fact that there are few, if any, who have the complete expertise in all of the fields of science required to deal with each step of material development and clinical testing. With this realization, or possibly rationalization, this author has only attempted to provide a general picture of some of the difficulties as well as necessary conditions required in the development of polymeric biomaterials. This objective will be pursued by first directing attention to some general considerations of polymeric biomedical systems (Pt. II) followed by a more detailed discussion of the chemical and material characteristics of polyurethane systems as an example (Pt. III). Part IV attempts to provide a brief overview of some of the areas where the urethane systems have been

medically applied as well as some of the difficulties encountered
in their clinical testing. The realization that many of the difficulties encountered are a function of material composition or fabrication has prompted the author to again state that the need to know
or be aware of as much of the complete implant development as
possible is crucial for the development of a successful implant
material.

II. SOME BASIC CONSIDERATIONS OF POLYMER SYSTEMS

Since the subject of this book is heavily concerned with applications of synthetic polymers as biomaterials, one might first
take a moment to focus on the polymeric makeup of the physiological system. In doing so, we realize each one of us is a living
organized mass of polymeric substances with some additional and
essential additives and fillers, as water, lipids, electrolytes,
etc. Clearly the most abundant polymeric material would be collagen, one of the structural proteins of high content in connective
tissue, bone, and the vascular system. Some other proteins in
this same category include elastin, keratin, reticulin, myosin,
and actin, the latter two being prime components of muscle. In
contrast to the structural proteins, there is an excessive number
of globular proteins or enzymes. These have no major mechanical
function, but rather serve as the biological catalysts to sustain
the metabolic processes of life. The significant point is that both
groups of proteins are derived from the basic twenty plus amino
acids and, by "control" of the polymeric nucleic acids DNA, RNA,
etc., these building blocks or monomer units are bound together
to provide a polymer or macromolecule with a specific function.
The basic polymerization scheme can be illustrated as:

$$
\begin{array}{c}
\overset{H}{\underset{H}{\diagdown}}\kern-2pt N - \overset{\overset{\displaystyle H}{|}}{\underset{\underset{\displaystyle R_1}{|}}{C}} - \overset{\displaystyle O}{C\diagup\diagdown}\kern-2pt OH \;+\; \overset{H}{\underset{H}{\diagdown}}\kern-2pt N - \overset{\overset{\displaystyle H}{|}}{\underset{\underset{\displaystyle R_2}{|}}{C}} - \overset{\displaystyle O}{C\diagup\diagdown}\kern-2pt OH \;\longrightarrow
\end{array}
$$

$$
\overset{H}{\underset{H}{\diagdown}}N - \overset{\overset{H}{|}}{\underset{\underset{R_1}{|}}{C}} - \overset{O}{\overset{\|}{C}} - N - \overset{\overset{H}{|}}{\underset{\underset{R_2}{|}}{C}} - C\diagup\diagdown OH \;+\; H_2O
$$

(A)

$$
(A) \;+\; \overset{H}{\underset{H}{\diagdown}}N - \overset{\overset{H}{|}}{\underset{\underset{R_3}{|}}{C}} - C\diagup\diagdown OH \;\longrightarrow
$$

$$
\overset{H}{\underset{H}{\diagdown}}N - \overset{\overset{H}{|}}{\underset{\underset{R_1}{|}}{C}} - \overset{O}{\overset{\|}{C}} - N - \overset{\overset{H}{|}}{\underset{\underset{R_2}{|}}{C}} - \overset{O}{\overset{\|}{C}} - N - \overset{\overset{H}{|}}{\underset{\underset{R_3}{|}}{C}} - C\diagup\diagdown OH \;+\; H_2O
$$

This results in a linear polymer chain with a repeat unit of

$$
\{\overset{\overset{H}{|}}{N} - \overset{\overset{O}{\|}}{C} - \overset{\overset{H}{|}}{\underset{\underset{R}{|}}{C}}\} \quad \text{where the composition of R is dependent on the type}
$$

of amino acid, e.g., if glycine, R is hydrogen.

The difference between any two proteins, be they globular or structural, is in the type as well as the sequential arrangement of the amino acid residues. Specifically, the nature of the side group

R may be polar, nonpolar, large, or small and this affects the
degree of interaction between other groups of the same molecule
(intramolecular) or with different molecules (intermolecular). The

$$\begin{array}{cc} H & O \\ | & || \\ \end{array}$$

sequential arrangement of the basic amide (-N-C-) coupling is also
important in influencing the geometric conformation of the molecule, e.g., helical, coiled, etc. (Fig. 1). Many of these same arguments have general applicability to the polynucleic acids, DNA being the most important polymer and the essence of life. The mucopolysaccharides, such as heparin, hyaluronic acid, or chondroitin
sulfate, also have their molecular conformation influenced by the
nature of the repeat unit as well as the sequential arrangement of
these units. Molecular conformation is an essential consideration,
for it may control whether the macromolecule can pack with others
in an ordered fashion, e.g., in a crystalline lattice as may occur
with collagen, keratin, or numerous other proteins (both globular
and structural), polynucleic acids, and mucopolysaccharides.
This intermolecular packing may be essential for the function of
the molecule, e.g., in building an ordered tissue such as striated
muscle. It may be of little importance in other situations as in a
monomolecular enzyme. The significant point, however, is that

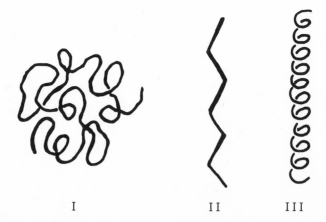

I   II   III

FIGURE 1. Schematic showing simplified sketches of possible
molecular conformations: I) random coil; II) extended planar
zigzag chain; III) helical chain.

from a limited number of building blocks or monomers, nature has developed an incredible variety of polymeric macromolecules that control nearly all of our physiological processes. Because of this, one might be sparked to consider whether, in the quest for biomaterial systems, one should attempt to utilize these same building blocks. While there is no confirmed answer to this question, it is reasonable to say that not all biomaterial problems would be solved by this approach, that is, natural regeneration which occurs in a physiological system would not occur in an implant. While the future possibility for stimulated regeneration is an impetus to this approach, it is reasonable that other building blocks and, therefore, new macromolecules will have to be developed, particularly for long-term application. This statement does not rule out the chemical modification of naturally occurring polymers, e.g., modified reconstituted collagen, elastin, etc.

In accepting the fact that other polymeric materials are needed for biomaterial application, questions arise as to the criteria upon which the most suitable polymer composition can be designed chemically. Unfortunately, at this time, these criteria are not available although some significant advances have been made in the last decade. As is the general case, the need has spurred the scientific approach to find these criteria. That is, off-the-shelf commercial stock polymers were first utilized, and in some cases still are, for various biomaterial applications for lack of other more standardized and characterized materials. The principal criteria initially used were mainly based on information obtained outside of a physiological system, for example, mechanical properties, chemical inertness, solubility or swelling in water, etc. Only in recent years, and only after material failure leading to death in many cases, has attention been given to more subtle phenomena such as lipid absorption, surface free energy, zeta potential behavior, long-term creep or fatigue properties, chemical purity and fabrication history.

To appreciate the problems with off-the-shelf commercial polymers that were developed without intent for biomedical applications, we need only point out a few basic facts. First, the state of chemical purity is of extreme importance. Coupled to this is the fact that even a given polymer is not necessarily made by the same chemical route. That is, different chemical routes can be used in the polymerization of polyethylene, polyurethane, etc., but these can result in differences in catalyst residue levels and type as well as monomer or oligomer concentration, let alone

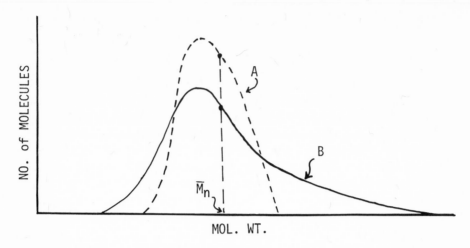

FIGURE 2. Two hypothetical molecular weight distributions illustrating very different breadths yet having the same number average (mean) molecular weight indicated by $\overline{M}n$.

different molecular weight distributions. Some examples of this
will be made apparent later when discussing the chemistry of polyurethanes in Part III. This point of trace catalyst or other impurities is emphasized since it may be this residue which triggers
thrombus formation, protein deposition, giant cell growth or other
unfavorable tissue responses in actual application while the basic
polymer may have been satisfactory or tissue compatible. Even
more significant is an awareness of whether any fillers such as
talc, carbon black, etc., or additives such as antioxidants or stabilizers are present, and if so, what kind and what level of content.
Also, as stated above different chemical routes can lead to the
same basic polymer but may result in different molecular weight
distribution although the average molecular weight may be the
same. This point is also important for the material properties
are in many ways affected by this distribution. Specifically, low
molecular weight species tend to make the material less viscous
or less resistant to flow whereas a high molecular weight tail in
the distribution helps to resist flow (Fig. 2).

With respect to biomaterial considerations, one of the most significant material properties associated with the molecular weight distribution is creep, i.e., the time dependence of strain (change in length) under a given load. It must be remembered, however, that comparison of molecular weights or their distribution for two different polymers as polyethylene with a polyurethane, is generally meaningless. This is because the viscoelastic behavior of a given polymer type also depends on chain conformation, flexibility and inter- and intramolecular forces. Using our example, we note that polyethylene possesses only van der Waals' intermolecular forces whereas the typical polyurethanes can have considerably stronger intermolecular forces due to hydrogen bonding as discussed in Part III. Nylon (polyamides) and protein (polypeptides) are other examples of strong hydrogen bonding systems.

Finally, the fabrication history may be of great importance with respect to final application. Factors such as degree of crystallinity, phase separation, molecular orientation and surface texture may be significant in terms of use properties. Many of these factors relate not only to mechanical properties (modulus, fatigue, creep, etc.), but also to other significant biomaterial considerations such as surface free energy (wetting), refractive index and tissue ingrowth or adherence, etc. With proper methodology, these parameters can be controlled. Direct examples of this will be illustrated in the next section where some detail is given to a discussion of the chemical and physical aspects of polyurethane materials. It might be pointed out that, while this discussion will focus on urethane systems, many of the same considerations alluded to are of prime importance in dealing with other biomaterial problems occurring with other types of polymers.

III. POLYURETHANES

With the exception of many of the natural polymers, those that have been produced synthetically have been in existence a relatively short time. This is the case for polyurethanes which were first produced in 1937 by Bayer and co-workers [1]. Since that date, a whole field of urethane chemistry has evolved and is now at the point where the order of one billion pounds of polyurethanes are produced annually.

The types of materials fabricated from these systems are great and extend from the area of coatings to large molded devices.

One of the largest volume items is foam materials. It is quite safe to say that at this time, polyurethane-based biomaterials are a very small fraction of the urethane market. While this is no surprise, it is a significant point for it limits the number of pure or biomedical urethane-based materials available to the medical profession, a related industry*. In general, this is true for most polymeric biomaterials, with some exceptions such as various silicone polymers as the well-known Silastic materials. The reason for this lack of a wide variety of biomedical grade polymeric materials is simple: it would be a low-volume business for the majority of the polymer producing industries. This means a high investment but low return for these companies. Fortunately, however, with considerable contract support through NIH and particularly the materials program of the National Heart and Lung Institute, much of the fundamental research costs are being absorbed, thereby stimulating the development of more and better materials suitable for implantation. Should this effort continue, we will hopefully see scientific biomaterial reports concerned with commercial off-the-shelf items disappear and those utilizing well characterized materials begin to be the standard.

Urethane Chemistry

In general, urethane chemistry is but a branch of isocyanate chemistry. The impetus for Bayer to utilize this technology was the hope of developing synthetic polymeric materials that were elastomeric and that could compete with natural rubber systems.

Since there are books written on urethanes and isocyanate chemistry alone [2, 3, 4, 5, 6], we will only introduce some of the basic characteristics of the synthetic schemes used in preparing urethane polymers and in particular those urethane systems which are referred to as segmented**. These are emphasized since the majority of the urethane biomaterials being investigated today are of this type.

---

*Possibly one of the most well developed biomedical grade of polyurethane available today is that obtainable from Ethicon, Inc. under the tradename of Biomer.

**Segmented refers to the general class of polyurethanes which have chains made of alternating sequences of flexible (soft segment - SS) and rigid stiff (hard segment - HS) units.

Chain formation is brought about by first reacting a flexible macrodiol (a) with an excess of diisocyanate (b) to produce a

macrodiisocyanate (c) with urethane linkages $\left(N - C - O \right)$ (with H and O shown above the N–C)

$$HO \sim\!\!\sim\!\!\sim OH + OCN-R-NCO \rightarrow OCN-R-N-C-O \sim\!\!\sim\!\!\sim O-C-N-R-NCO$$

      (a)   (b)   (c)

In practice, a homologous mixture of short chain polymeric diiso-cyanates is produced in this reaction; however, the distribution is dependent upon the relative stoichiometry, temperature and re-action kinetics of the specific diisocyanate and diol. The macro-diisocyanate (c) can then be reacted with more diol to produce a linear polymer chain or chain extension may be carried out by re-acting (c) with a low molecular weight diol or a diamine $(H_2N\text{-}R\text{-}NH_2)$. A three-step process is illustrated below where an additional capping step is added (Step II) for the purpose of mini-mizing hard segment distribution size [7].

Step I : Capping of a macrodiol (a) with diisocyanate (b).

$$HO \sim\!\!\sim\!\!\sim OH + OCN-R_1-NCO \rightarrow OCN-R_1 \sim\!\!\sim\!\!\sim\!\!\sim R_1-NCO$$

       (a)   (b)   (c)

                 (excess)

Step II : Double capping of part of the above product with a diamine (d).

$$c + H_2N-R_2-NH_2 \rightarrow H_2N-R_2 \sim\!\!\sim\!\!\sim R_2NH_2$$

               (d)

            (excess)

Step III: Chain extension

$$OCN-R_1 \sim\!\!\sim\!\!\sim R_1NCO + H_2N-R_2 \sim\!\!\sim\!\!\sim R_2-NH_2 \rightarrow \text{Polyurethane}$$

The preceding scheme is a three-step process, but it is also
possible to use a one-step process by varying the stoichiometry
and adding the chain-extending diamine or diol in the first step.
Another common modification is to use water as a chain extender
which results in the off-gassing of carbon dioxide producing urea

$$
\begin{array}{ccc}
H & O & H \\
| & || & | \\
\end{array}
$$

linkages $\{N - C - N\}$ as shown below [8, 9].

$$OCN \,\sim\sim\, NCO + OCN \,\sim\sim\, NCO + H_2O \;\rightarrow$$

$$OCN\{\sim\sim\sim NH{-}CO{-}NH\sim\sim\sim NHCO{-}NH\sim\sim\sim\}NCO + CO_2$$

This is a particularly useful route when producing foam materials.

Depending on the synthetic route, a one-, two-, or even a
three-step process, the final polymer makeup will vary accordingly, i.e., in diol content, etc. This, of course, will be reflected in property behavior. Also, the low molecular weight species and/or residue oligomeric ingredients incorporated or resid-
ing in the reaction vessel or precipitated polymer may well be important, particularly in biomaterial applications where pure polymers may be required.

While the above introduction to urethane polymerization is
brief, one realizes that in the final solid state of these materials,
the intermolecular forces may be considerable due to the presence
of hydrogen bonding [10, 11, 12]. This is schematically illustrated
in Figure 3. While these forces tend to promote intermolecular
attraction, there generally is thermodynamic incompatibility of
the HS and SS regions such that microphase separation or domain
formation may occur as depicted in Figure 4 [13]. Due to the
glassy, paracrystalline or crystalline character of the HS, the HS
domains serve as pseudocrosslinks to help minimize flow in the
system when deformed. Furthermore, the mechanical properties
can be varied accordingly, depending on the degree of HS content,
domain formation, and its character. That is, for a given set of
ingredients, the relative content of the HS and SS material can be
varied, and will markedly affect the stress strain behavior as
shown by an example series of segmented polyurethanes in Figure
5. As is obvious, the SS is so named for it is designed to be
rubberlike or "soft" at the use temperature of the material, i.e.,

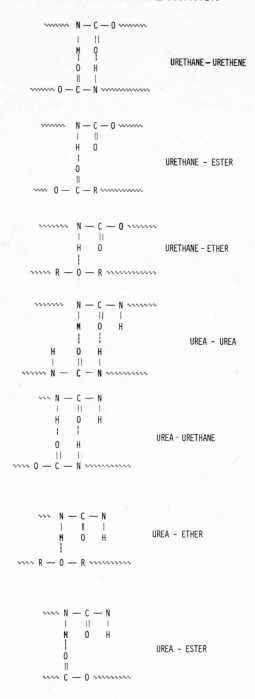

FIGURE 3. Possible types of hydrogen bonding that commonly occur in polyurethane systems.

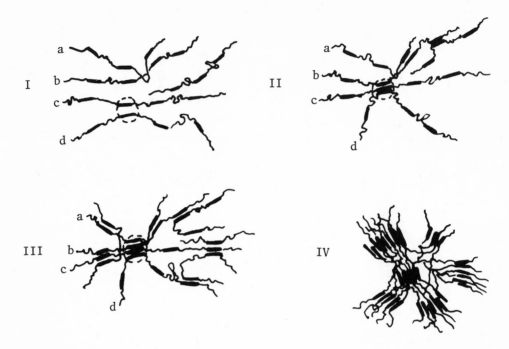

FIGURE 4. Schematic of the formation of domain structure in
segmented polyurethanes. Dark heavy lines represent the hard
segments; the lighter lines represent the soft segments.

its respective glass transition temperature, T_g, is below the use
temperature. By varying the type of macrodiol used, this T_g can
be controlled. Not only can T_g be altered, but the chemical makeup of the SS is very significant with respect to HS compatibility.
Therefore, the chemical composition can influence domain formation and, hence, properties. For example, if a polyester SS is
used, the ester carbonyl is available for strong hydrogen bonding
with the conventional HS containing amide hydrogen*. This is in

---

*It is possible to prepare HS material without the presence of
hydrogen bonding [15].

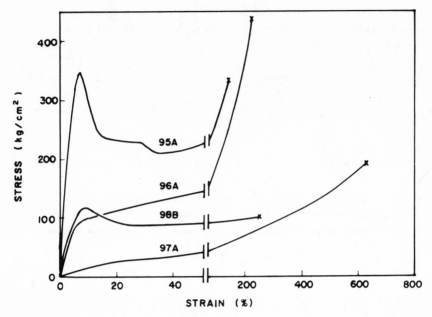

FIGURE 5. Stress strain behavior for a systematic series of segmented urethanes made from polyethylene glycol, 4,4'-dicyclo-
hexylmethane diisocyanate and p-phenylene diamine. The soft
segment content for the series is 95A (27%), 96A (53%), 97A (68%),
98B (88%); [19].

contrast to a polyether SS where the degree of hydrogen bonding
to the ether linkage is decreased and the bonding is weaker.

The SS may also be chosen so that it can crystallize once the
polymer is oriented. This can be a reversible process as it is in
natural rubber and can be advantageous in certain material applications where viscous flow at high deformation is undesirable
and/or where high tensile strength is desirable [14].

In many segmented urethanes, the SS homopolymer may crystallize quiescently. This is minimized or eliminated in the corresponding segmented systems due to the short lengths of the SS
as well as the diluent effects caused by the presence of the HS
material [15]. Should SS crystallization occur, however, the
properties are markedly and generally undesirably affected. An
example of this behavior occurs in Figure 5 with sample 98 where
the molecular weight of the soft segment was high enough and of

sufficient content to lead to SS crystallization. Clearly the modulus and overall stress strain behavior is greatly changed from
that of sample number 97.

Some of the many types of hard and soft segments, diiso-
cyanates and chain extenders are shown in Table I. While each of
these may be incorporated into a polymer termed a polyurethane

due to the presence of the urethane linkage ($-N-C-O-$), it is clear

$$\begin{array}{cc} H & O \\ | & || \\ -N - C & - O- \end{array}$$

from the previous discussion that the chemical composition can
vary tremendously. Furthermore, Table I shows but a small number of the possible ingredients. For example, no consideration
has been given to crosslinked urethanes produced by incorporating
a trifunctional unit such as a triol or triamine as shown below.
Sulfur vulcanization can also be carried out if one of the ingredients possesses one or more double bonds [9].

$$H_2N-R_1 \sim\!\!\sim R_1-NH_2 + HO \sim\!\!\sim OH + R_2(OH)_3$$

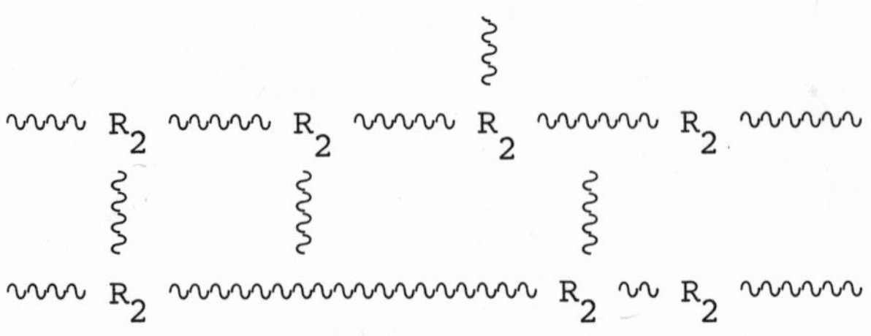

crosslinked insoluble network

Also, we have avoided discussion dealing with the many possible
side reactions that can occur during urethane polymerization.
Two common examples of these are shown in the following and concern the so-called biuret and allophanate formation:

Biuret Formation:

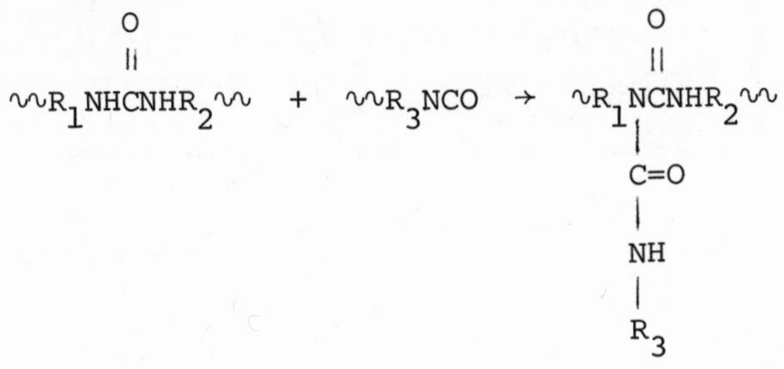

$$\underset{\|}{\overset{O}{}}\sim\sim R_1 NHCNHR_2 \sim\sim \quad + \quad \sim\sim R_3 NCO \quad \rightarrow \quad \sim R_1 \underset{|}{\overset{O}{\overset{\|}{}}} NCNHR_2 \sim\sim$$

$$C=O$$
$$|$$
$$NH$$
$$|$$
$$R_3$$

Allophanate Formation:

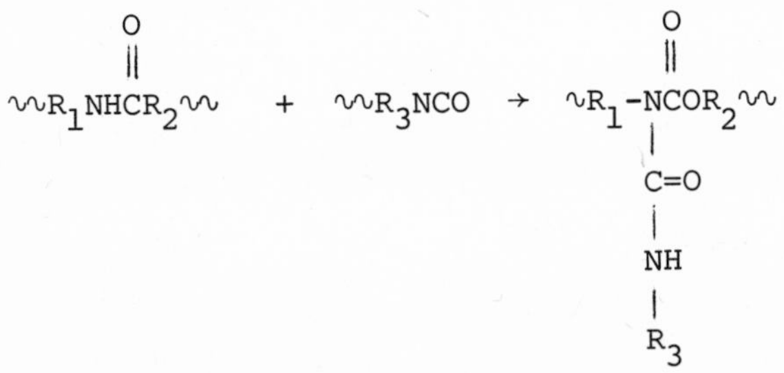

$$\overset{O}{\underset{\|}{}}\sim\sim R_1 NHCR_2 \sim\sim \quad + \quad \sim\sim R_3 NCO \quad \rightarrow \quad \sim R_1 \overset{O}{\underset{\|}{}} -NCOR_2 \sim\sim$$

$$C=O$$
$$|$$
$$NH$$
$$|$$
$$R_3$$

The point of illustrating these two possible side reactions is to emphasize again that a given polyurethane may contain other than the usual urethane or urea linkages. Therefore, when a given ure-thane is found to be a "poor" or "good" biomaterial, one must not be too quick to disqualify the general class of urethanes but must consider the detailed composition as well as the preparative con-ditions.

Structure, Morphology, and Properties

As alluded to above, the urethanes may give rise to consider-able hydrogen bonding (Fig. 3) and to domain structure (Fig. 4). More homogeneous structures can also occur if the ingredients are compatible. In crosslinked systems, the homogeneity in structure may also be controlled by when the crosslinking is carried out and by the nature of the crosslinking agent. Higher, super order mole-cular structure can also be induced as has been illustrated by Wilkes, et al. [16, 17, 18, 19, 20, 21]. For example, it has been illustrated by the author and co-workers that a large anisotropic

TABLE I

EXAMPLE INGREDIENTS FOR THE PREPARATION OF
SEGMENTED POLYURETHANES

	Diisocyanates
Name	Structure

Diphenylmethane diisocyanate (MDI)

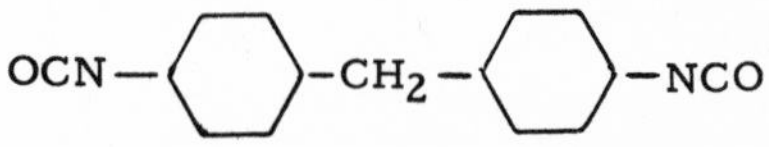

$OCN-\langle\bigcirc\rangle-CH_2-\langle\bigcirc\rangle-NCO$

Tolylene diisocyanate (TDI)

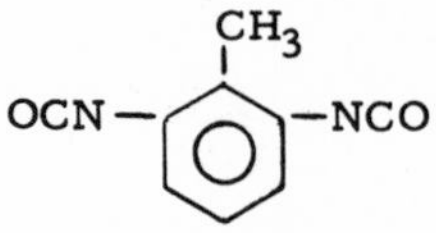

CH$_3$ CH$_3$
$OCN-\bigcirc-NCO$ $\bigcirc-NCO$
                                      NCO
2,6-TDI   2,4-TDI

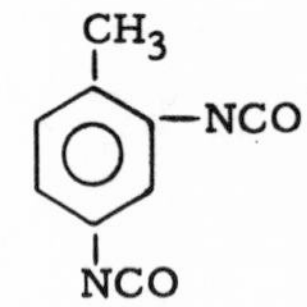

Tolidine diisocyanate (TODI)

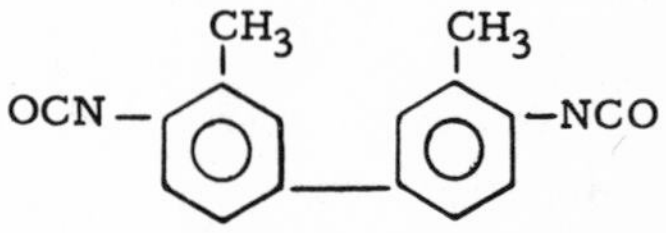

CH$_3$ CH$_3$
$OCN-\bigcirc-\bigcirc-NCO$

Xylylene diisocyanate (XDI)

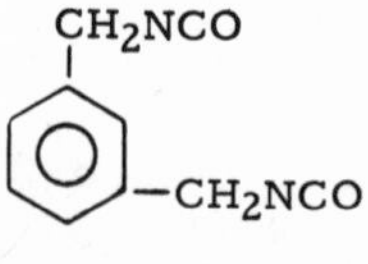

CH$_2$NCO
$\bigcirc-CH_2NCO$

4,4'-Dicyclohexylmethane-
   diisocyanate (Hylene W)

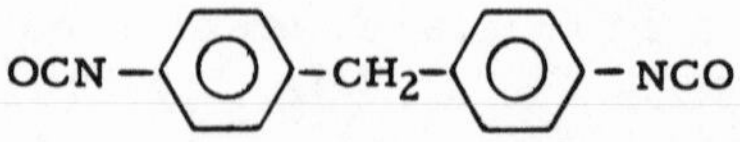

$OCN-\langle\bigcirc\rangle-CH_2-\langle\bigcirc\rangle-NCO$

TABLE I (Cont.)

| | Macrodiols* |
Name	Structure
Hydroxyl-terminated poly-ethylene oxide**	$HO-CH-CH_2 \left(\!+O-CH_2-CH_2\!\right)_x OH$
Hydroxyl-terminated poly-propylene oxide**	$HO-CH_2-\overset{\overset{\displaystyle CH_3}{\vert}}{CH}\left(\!+O-CH_2-\overset{\overset{\displaystyle CH_3}{\vert}}{CH}\!\right)_x OH$
Hydroxyl-terminated tetra-methylene oxide**	$HO-(CH_2)_4\left(\!+O\,[\,CH_2]_4\!\right)_x OH$
Copolymer of the above two systems (sequence distribution of ethylene oxide and propylene oxide may vary)	$HO\left(\!+[\,CH_2]_2-O\!\right)_x\left(\!+CH_2-\overset{\overset{\displaystyle CH_3}{\vert}}{CH}-O\!\right)_y H$

---

*Only polyether diols shown; polyester diols are also commonly used.

**Note: x is generally within the range of 8-40.

TABLE I (Cont.)

Diamines
(will provide urea linkages)

Name	Structure

Ortho (1), meta (2), and para (3) phenylene diamine

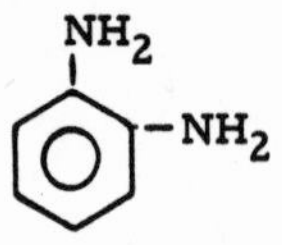

Benzidine

$$H_2N-\langle O \rangle-\langle O \rangle-NH_2$$

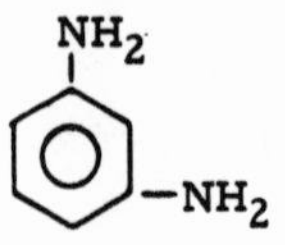

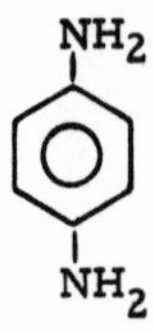

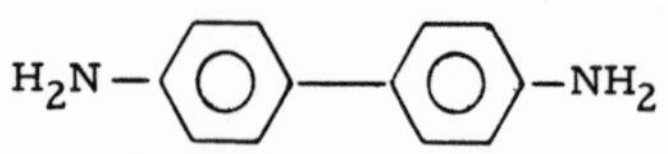

Methylene-bis-o-chloroaniline (MOCA)

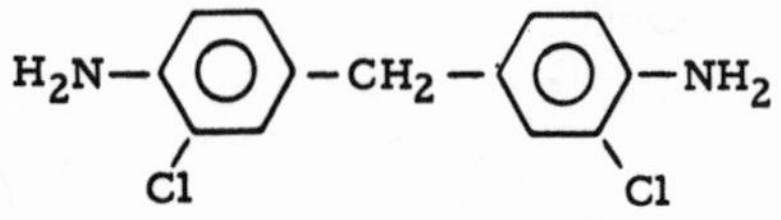

$$H_2N-\langle O \rangle-CH_2-\langle O \rangle-NH_2$$
$$\qquad\quad Cl \qquad\qquad\quad Cl$$

p, p'-Diaminediphenyl methane

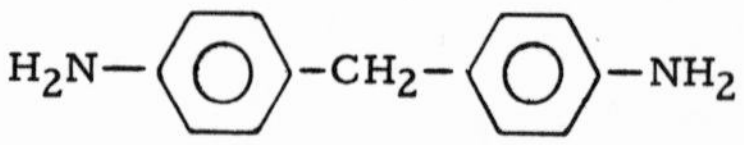

$$H_2N-\langle O \rangle-CH_2-\langle O \rangle-NH_2$$

1, 2-Diaminopropane

$$\qquad\qquad\qquad CH_3$$
$$H_2N-CH_2-CH-NH_2$$

Ethylene diamine

$$H_2N-CH_2-CH_2-NH_2$$

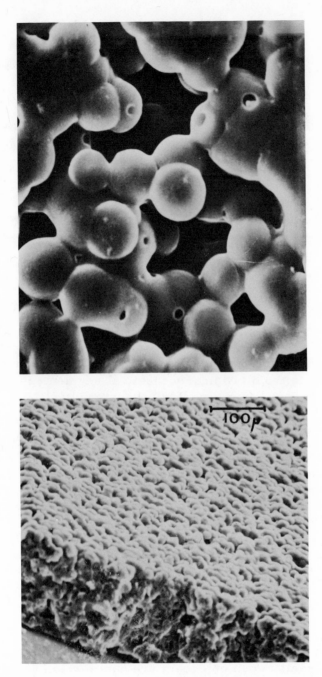

FIGURE 6. Scanning electron micrographs of a solution cast film of a nonhydrogen bonding polyether segmented urethane. Note the porosity between spherulites [16].

N1 : N4 MIXTURES

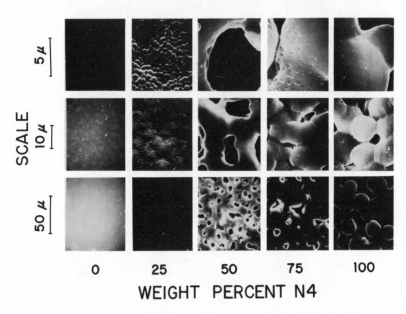

FIGURE 7. Scanning electron micrographs of a series of solution cast films made from two nearly identical segmented urethanes. Note the great range in morphological texture [17].

spherulitic structure can be induced (Fig. 6). In fact, by using well characterized polymers with known systematic structure, unique porous films could be produced as shown in Figure 7. It has recently been verified that similar spherulitic structure has been noted in more conventional segmented materials [19, 20, 22]. While the details of this spherulitic structure have little need to be discussed in this paper, the significant point is that the gross structure of the material can be controlled in many instances. This means factors such as surface roughness and porosity can be varied. Clearly, this control may be useful in biomaterial applications, e.g., where cellular ingrowth is desirable. Related to this latter application, it may be possible to develop open cell foam urethanes which could be of value for tissue scaffolding. possible to develop open cell foam urethanes which could be of value for tissue scaffolding.

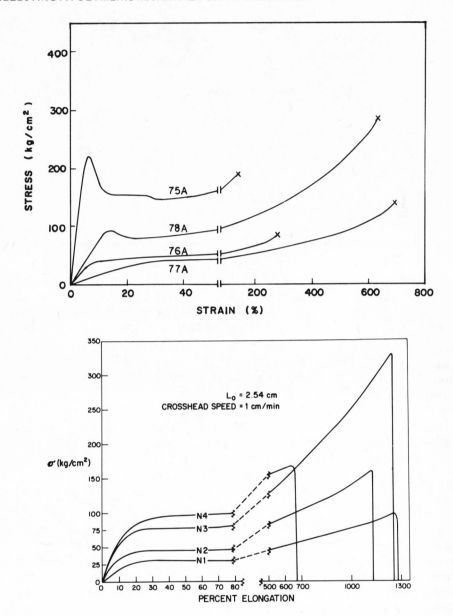

FIGURE 8. Two series of stress strain curves for two very different series of segmented urethanes. A) This series is essentially identical with that shown in Figure 5 except for the fact that ethylene diamine was used in place of p-phenylene diamine. B) These data were obtained from a systematic series of nonhydrogen bonding segmented urethanes shown in Figure 8C.

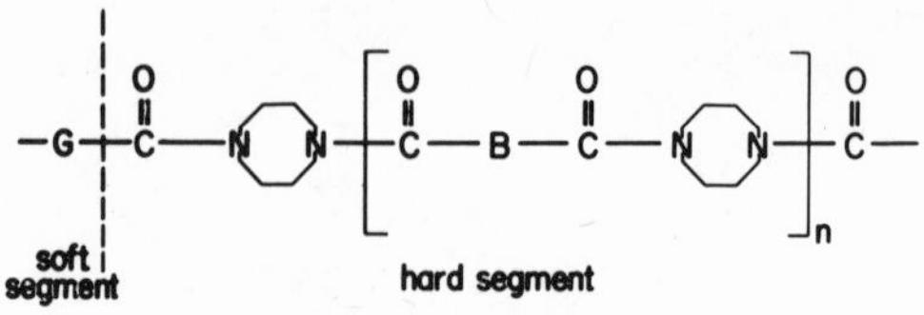

G = $+OCH_2CH_2CH_2CH_2\}_{\overline{137}}O-$

B = $+OCH_2CH_2CH_2CH_2\}-O-$

n = 1, 2, 3, 4

FIGURE 8C

To generalize the properties of polyurethanes is clearly not readily possible for, as already shown by Figure 5, even a given series of segmented urethanes varies drastically in stress strain behavior. This is again illustrated in Figures 8A and 8B for two other characterized series of segmented systems. The series shown in Figure 8A is identical to that in Figure 5 with the exception that a different diamine was used. Figure 8B, however, is a series where no hydrogen bonding is present and where the hard segment sizes are monodisperse.

In many biomaterial applications, it may be desirable to be able to fabricate or mold the implant piece at the time of implantation. With many of the segmented polyurethanes, one must therefore be aware of any time-dependent effects in the stabilization of properties following fabrication. It has been only recently that initial time-dependent properties have been noted by the author and co-workers [23]. Figure 9A shows one example of the time-dependence of modulus for a commercial urethane following heat treatment (as molding). Figure 9B shows the corresponding calorimetric scans on the same material. It is apparent that (a) there is a significant change in modulus over the first three hours, and (b) the thermal properties are also very time-dependent. Without going into detail on this example or the other urethanes that were studied, this behavior can be accounted for on the basis of the time dependence of HS domain formation and its thermal stability in a given system. Similar studies on other urethane systems have shown even more drastic time-dependent changes.

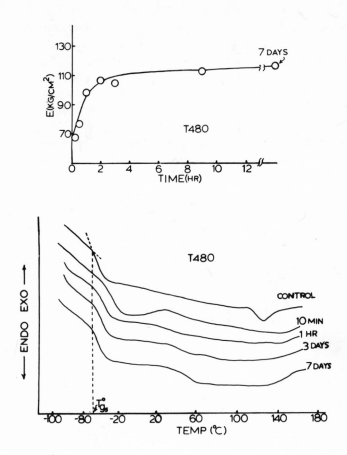

FIGURE 9. A) Young's modulus and B) DSC thermogram traces
for a typical segmented urethane (Texin 480-A).   The different
times represent the time after the sample had been rapidly
quenched from 170°C to room temperature.

Since apparently this time-dependent phenomenon has been overlooked until now, it suggests that property data reported on segmented urethanes may be meaningless on an absolute basis unless some knowledge of the testing time, storage temperature, etc., is given, i.e., complete material history.

In general, all the urethane systems are viscoelastic materials and this should not be overlooked in material applications. Figure 10 illustrates this characteristic nature of these materials where the stress strain behavior of a commercial segmented urethane is shown for the initial and the fifth deformation cycle. One notes that (a) the recovery curve for the first cycle displays considerable hysteresis, and (b) the deformation behavior of the fifth cycle shows that the material has softened considerably as compared to the initial loading. This softening effect and hysteresis behavior may be of importance in material application where cyclic

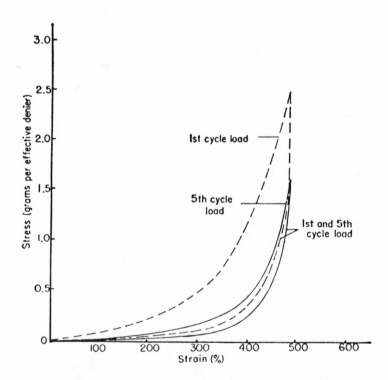

FIGURE 10.   Typical stress strain behavior for a segmented urethane fiber.   Effective denier is the denier at the point of measurement [8].

loading is required. Such behavior can be accounted for as the basis of HS domain breakdown and their rearrangement or orientation. In fact, with respect to orientation, it has been found that the HS and SS material orients differently under an applied strain. It has also been shown that following release of strain after deformation, the SS material generally recovers (disorients) to a much higher degree than do the HS domains [24, 25]. Thus, increasing HS content may increase strength, but it generally leads to a less elastomeric material. Upon deformation, there is rearrangement of hydrogen bonding which can also help to stabilize the deformed structure and, hence, increase permanent set behavior [26].

Although not displayed in Figure 10, the deformation rate or deformation frequency is also of prime importance with respect to the molecular relaxation rates of a polymer system. These relaxation rates are in turn controlled by such fundamental parameters as polymer type, molecular weight distribution, degree of crystallinity, domain structure, etc. Hence, it is strictly fortuitous to find a suitable material for a specific biomaterial application without regard to the above fundamental parameters. It is also realized that in the case of a material application where the deformation behavior is complex, simple deformation data may not provide sufficient information with respect to in situ behavior. There is little doubt, however, that depending on the application, certain fundamental data or characterization data can be of considerable value in helping to select the right material. While this last point cannot be overemphasized, it should also be stated that the choice of the kind of fundamental information required is not always obvious and caution must be taken not to waste man hours in gathering interesting but useless data.

In the fabrication of a biomaterial device, there are generally one or more "polymer processing" steps. While the laboratory scale fabrication may indicate the successful development of a suitable biomaterial device, once the production becomes scaled up, new problems may arise. These can originate from many sources. Impurities may result in the material through the use of mold release agents, machine oil, or possible chemical degradation due to excessive temperatures or long processing resonance times. Metallic fragments in the material may result from natural machine abrasion during a processing operation as grinding, compounding or mixing, or extrusion. Also, the chemical nature of the polymer may be modified through surface oxidation caused by high processing temperatures. In some cases, these thermally induced chemical changes can lead to crosslinking reactions or to chain scission. Either effect results in molecular weight changes that can influence the material properties. While not wishing to belabor the processing aspects, since they may vary widely depending on each individual polymer type, it is readily apparent that the procedural details of the final fabrication should be carefully considered and monitored.

IV. POLYURETHANES AS BIOMATERIALS

A survey of the biomaterial literature quickly reveals that a considerable number of papers have been published which deal with the in vivo or in vitro evaluation of polyurethanes. There also have been a variety of biomaterial devices constructed from these base polymers.

An indication of the diversity of the applications in which the urethanes have been utilized is obtained from the following list:

> Endotracheal tubes [27]
> Aortic grafts [28]
> Arterial, venous or vascular tubing [29, 30, 31]
> Heart assist or heart bypass devices [30, 31, 32, 33, 34]
> Dialysis membranes [35, 36]
> Artificial heart chambers [32, 33]
> Pacemaker wire insulation
> Heart valves [37, 38]
> Bone adhesives [39, 40]
> Cavity liners in dentures [39]
> Breast augmentation
> Splint devices [39]
> Preventive and restorative dentistry [39, 41]
> Roller pump tubing in artificial heart or blood pumps
> [34, 42, 43)

While the preceding list is indeed impressive with respect to the range of applications, not all of these were found entirely satisfactory as will be noted in some of the corresponding references.

However, as stated shortly, an unsuccessful application may be misleading with respect to the failure of the basic polymer used.

While the list gives direct biomaterial utilization, other studies have considered the direct consideration of tissue response [44, 45, 46, 47, 48, 49], chemical biodegradation [32, 42, 45, 48, 49, 50], hydrolytic stability [43, 51], time-dependent property changes in vivo [32, 38, 48], and blood compatibility of heparinized, unheparinized and carbon black-modified systems [31, 32, 52, 53, 54, 55]. Consideration of texture (porosity) for specific applications has also been briefly investigated [55].

Many of the results of these direct device or compatibility evaluations must be taken with extreme caution. This is also true for those reports dealing with in vitro or in vivo studies as tissue response, tissue or cell culture tests or even blood compatibility. The reason for this suggested caution is two-fold and holds not just for urethane materials, but essentially for all types of bio-materials. First, many of the materials discussed are uncharac-terized in terms of chemical composition, let alone trace effects of impurities. This simply means that failure of a given material does not necessarily confirm that the basic polymer in the system is at fault, but only that, without further information, this par-ticular material or batch number (if commercial) is unsatisfactory. Failure itself may have arisen from trace catalyst, stabilizers, or other additives. The second basis for caution is the lack of stan-dardized testing or evaluation schemes, variability in human judgment coupled with limited statistical data, and finally, possible variability in surgical techniques.

In conclusion, it should be readily apparent that, in general, the considerations necessary for a polymeric material destined for a given biomaterial application are typically of high complexity. This complexity extends from the necessity of coupling the exper-tise of the polymer chemist with that of the material engineer, histologist, surgeon, etc. In many cases, even if this expertise is combined through teamwork, many problems still confront us due to various limitations in our present understanding of the physiological system and its response mechanism to a foreign material. In spite of this complexity, however, it is only through continued teamwork research that the present inherent problems will be overcome. The challenge is before us and we must all share our individual knowledge if the successful development of new biomaterials is to be a reality.

REFERENCES

1.   Farbenfabriken Bayer A. G., British Patent 769,682 (1952).

2.   Bruins, P. F., Ed., Polyurethane Technology, Interscience Publishers, John Wiley and Sons, N. Y., 1969.

3.   Beist, J. M. and Gudgeon, H., Advances in Polyurethane Technology, Maclaren and Sons, London, 1969.

4.   Saunders, J. H. and Frisch, K. C., Polyurethanes: Chemistry and Technology, Parts I and II, High Polymers, Vol. 16, Interscience Publishers, John Wiley and Sons, N. Y., 1962.

5.   Sayigh, A.A.R., Ulrich, H., and Farrissey, W. J., Jr., in Condensation Monomers, J. K. Stille and T. W. Campbell, Eds., High Polymers, Vol. 27, Interscience Publishers, John Wiley and Sons, N. Y., 1972, p. 369.

6.   Phillips, L. N. and Parker, D.B.V., Polyurethanes, Iliffe Books, London, 1964.

7.   Chang, Y. J. and Wilkes, G. L., manuscript to be submitted for publication in J. Polym. Sci.

8.   Hicks, E. M., Jr., Ultec, A. J., and Drougas, J., Science, 147, 373 (1965).

9.   Buist, J. M., Crowley, G. P., and Lowe, A., Encyclopedia of Polymer Science and Technology, H. F. Mark and N. G. Gaylord, Eds., Interscience Publishers, John Wiley and Sons, N. Y., 1971, Vol. 15, p. 445.

10. Seymour, R. W., and Cooper, S. L., presented at the meeting of the Rubber Division of the American Chemical Society, Denver, Colorado, 1973.

11. MacKnight, W. J. and Yang, M., J. Polym. Sci., Polym. Symp., 42, 817 (1973).

12. Tanaka, T., Yokoyama, T., and Kaku, K., Mem. Fac. Eng., Kyushu Univ., 23, 113 (1963).

13. Samuels, S. L., Ph.D. Thesis, Princeton University, 1973.

14. Morbitzer, L. and Hespe, H., J. Appl. Polym. Sci., 16, 2697 (1972).

15. Horrell, L. L., Macromolecules, 2, 607 (1969).

16. Samuels, S. L. and Wilkes, G. L., J. Polym. Sci., Polym. Symp., 43, 149 (1973).

17. Wilkes, G. L. and Samuels, S. L., J. Biomed. Mater. Res., 7, 541 (1973).

18. Wilkes, G. L., Samuels, S. L., and Crystal, R., J. Macromol. Sci., Phys. (in press).

19. Chang, Y. J., Wilkes, G. L., and Chen, C. T., Amer. Chem. Soc., Div. Polym. Chem., Prepr., 14, 1277 (1973).

20. Chang, Y. J., Ph.D. Thesis, Princeton University, 1974.

21. Wilkes, G. L. and Samuels, S. L., in Block and Graft Copolymers, J. Burke and V. Weiss, Eds., Syracuse University Press, Syracuse, N. Y., 1973, p. 225.

22. Desper, C. R., Illinger, J. L., and Schneider, N. S., Bull. Amer. Phys. Soc., March, 1974, paper BM3.

23. Wilkes, G. L., Bagrodia, S., Humphries, W., and Wildnauer, R., submitted to J. Polym. Sci., Polym. Lett. Ed.

24. Wilkes, G. L. and Samuels, S. L., in Block and Graft Copolymers, J. Burke and V. Weiss, Eds., Syracuse University Press, Syracuse, N. Y., 1973, p. 205.

25. Estes, G. M., Seymour, R. W., and Cooper, S. L., Macromolecules, 4, 452 (1972).

26. Wilkes, C. E. and Yusek, C., J. Macromol. Sci., Phys.,
     7, 157 (1973).

27. Boretos, J. W., Buttig, C. G., and Goodman, L., Anesth.
     Analg. (Cleveland), 51, 292 (1972).

28. Mirkovitch, V., Akutsu, T., and Kolff, W. J., Trans.
     Amer. Soc. Artif. Intern. Organs, 8, 79 (1962).

29. Wagner, M., Ruel, G., Teresi, J., and Kayser, K., Surg.,
     Gynecol., Obstet., 127, 805 (1968).

30. Kantrowitz, A., et al., Trans. Amer. Soc. Artif. Intern.
     Organs, 14, 344 (1968).

31. Boretos, J. W. and Pierce, W. S., Science, 158, 1481
     (1967).

32. Boretos, J. W., Pierce, W. S., Baier, R. E., Le Roy,
     A. F., and Donachy, H. J., presented at the 77th National
     Meeting of the American Institute of Chemical Engineers,
     Pittsburgh, Pa., May-June, 1974.

33. Pierce, W. S., Turner, M. C., Boretos, J. W., Nolan,
     S. P., and Morrow, A. G., Surgery, 66, 1034 (1969).

34. Kolobow, T., Zapol, W., and Pierce, J., Trans. Amer.
     Soc. Artif. Intern. Organs, 15, 172 (1969).

35. Lyman, D. J., and Loo, B. H., J. Biomed. Mater. Res.,
     1, 17 (1967).

36. Brauman, S. and Fritzinger, B., J. Appl. Polym. Sci.,
     16, 2439 (1972).

37. Hessel, E. A., May, K. J., Steinmetz, G. P., Jr.,
     Anderson, H. N., Dillard, D. H., and Merendino, K. A.,
     J. Thorac. Cardiov. Surg., 54, 227 (1967).

38. Boretos, J. W., Detmer, D. E., Donachy, J. H., and
     Mirkovitch, V., J. Biomed. Mater. Res., 5, 373 (1971).

39. Lee, H. and Neville, K., Handbook of Biomedical Plastics,
     Pasadena Technology Press, Pasadena, Calif., 1971.

40. Salvatore, J. E., Moncrief, W. H., Mandarino, M. P., and Sherman, R. T., Trans. Amer. Soc. Artif. Intern. Organs, 5, 325 (1960).

41. Patrick, R. L., et al., J. Dent. Res. 47, 12 (1968).

42. Boretos, J. W. and Pierce, W. S., J. Biomed. Mater. Res., 2, 121 (1965).

43. Boretos, J. W. and Wagner, F. R., ibid., 5, 411 (1971).

44. Rigdon, R. H., ibid., 7, 79 (1973).

45. Boretos, J. W., Proceedings of the 24th Annual Conference on Engineering in Medicine and Biology, Las Vegas, Nev., Vol. 13, 1971, p. 212.

46. Leininger, R. I., Amer. Soc. Test. Mater. Spec. Tech. Publ., No. 386, 71 (1968).

47. Lyman, D. J., Rev. Macromol. Chem., 1, 355 (1966).

48. Boretos, J. W., J. Biomed. Mater. Res., 6, 473 (1972).

49. Walter, J. C. and Chiaramonte, L. G., Brit. J. Surg., 52, 49 (1965).

50. Sherman, R. T. and Lyons, H., J. Surg. Res., 9, 167 (1969).

51. Cohen, J. L. and Van Aartsen, J. J., J. Polym. Sci., Polym. Symp., 42, 1325 (1973).

52. Sharp, W. V., Gardner, D. L., and Anderson, G. J., Trans. Amer. Soc. Artif. Intern. Organs, 12, 179 (1966).

53. Gardner, D. L., Sharp, W. V., Ewing, K. L., and Finelli, F., ibid., 15, 7 (1969).

54. Grode, G. A., Anderson, G. J., Grotta, N. M., and Falb, R. D., ibid., 15, 1 (1969).

55. Mirkovitch, V., et al., J. Appl. Physiol., 16, 381 (1961).

SURFACE-BONDED HEPARIN

R. D. Falb

Battelle, Columbus Laboratories
Columbus, Ohio 43201

The first report of surface-attached heparin was by Gott and co-workers in 1963 [1]. In this work, heparin was attached through formation of a complex with a quaternary ammonium salt which was adsorbed to graphite. The discovery of the thromboresistant properties of heparinized surfaces was inadvertent because the original intent of the work was to evaluate graphite. The graphite surface was treated with a quaternary ammonium salt to sterilize it, and the surface was rinsed in heparin as a simple precautionary measure. Gott's work showed that the marked thromboresistance of the graphite-benzalkonium-heparin (GBH) surface was due to the presence of heparin attached at the surface. This method held the promise of enabling one to use foreign surfaces in contact with blood without systemic anticoagulation. However, in practice, the GBH coating could not be applied to flexible materials, and thus its use was limited.

SYNTHESIS OF HEPARINIZED SURFACES

Shortly after Gott's work, a group at Battelle's Columbus Laboratories began a research program to develop methods of attaching heparin to the surfaces of a large number of synthetic and natural polymers. The goal of the research was to simply and rapidly bond heparin to materials such as silicone rubber, polyvinyl chloride, Teflon, and polyethylene which were in current use as blood-contacting materials. A second objective of the work was to determine the mechanism through which surface-bonded heparin inhibited clotting. The initial experimental approach to this work was the covalent attachment of a variety of quaternary ammonium salts to surfaces. Heparin bonding could then be effected on these surfaces by taking advantage of the ability of heparin to form highly nondissociable complexes with quaternary ammonium salts. The synthetic route taken in the initial stages of the work for the attachment of heparin was as follows [2]:

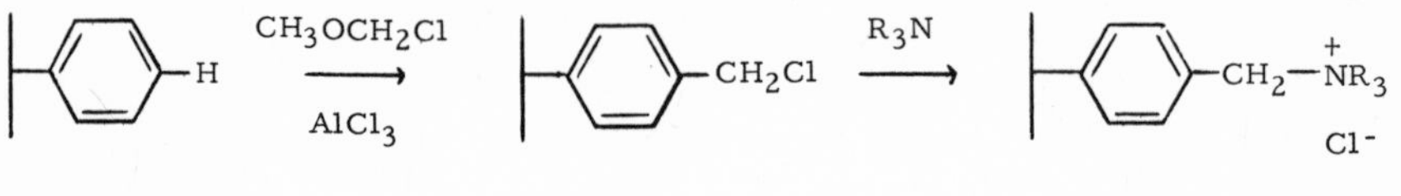

Polystyrene was selected as the first material for heparin attachment because of the ease with which it underwent electrophilic substitution at the surface. Since its properties were not suitable for implantation, procedures were then developed for heparinization of silicone rubber, polypropylene, polyethylene, and natural rubber by radiation grafting styrene to the surfaces of these materials. After grafting, the above sequence of reactions was performed to effect heparin binding.

A second, more direct route to attach heparin to polymer surfaces was achieved by radiation grafting of 4-vinyl pyridine or dimethylaminoethyl methacrylate to the surfaces as shown in the following reaction scheme [3]:

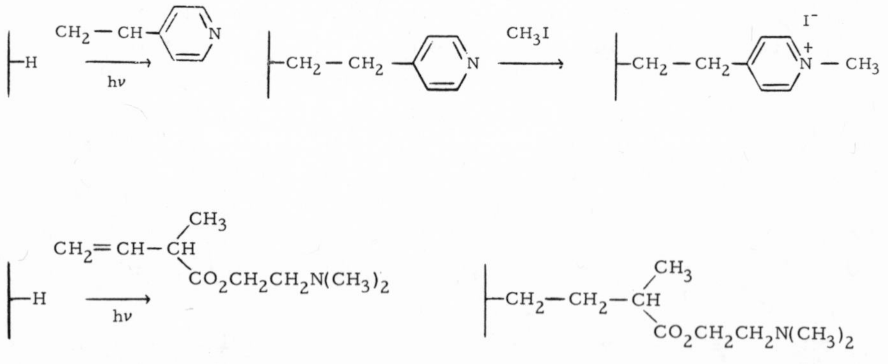

The above surface-bound quaternary ammonium salts complexed large amounts of heparin and had properties similar to those of the styrene-based surfaces.

A further method of attaching heparin involved the use of a plasticizer which contained amino groups. For example, polyvinyl chloride was plasticized by the addition of Hydrin rubber (a copolymer of epichlorohydrin and ethylene oxide which is then reacted with various monofunctional or difunctional amines.

An alternate route to heparinization of silicone rubber was developed in which the heparin binding site was attached to the silica filler. In this process, crosslinked silicone rubber was reacted with aminopropyltriethoxysilane to give a covalently attached amino group. This amine surface could be either further reacted with methyl iodide to effect quaternization or treated directly with heparin at a pH less than 7.0.

The methods discussed above resulted in varying amounts of bound heparin as determined by radioisotopic labeling techniques.

The effect of the attached heparin on thrombogenicity was evaluated in several ways. In an in vitro coagulation assay, recalcified blood in contact with a heparinized surface did not clot during a several-hour test period. When the blood was subsequently placed in a glass container, clotting occurred normally. The nonthrombogenicity of the surface as judged by this assay could not be related to the amount of heparin attached except that surfaces containing less than 1.0 μg/sq cm were thrombogenic. In some instances, surfaces with amounts of heparin as high as 5 μg/sq cm were thrombogenic, presumably because of nonhomogeneous coverage of the surface.

The covalent attachment of heparin to polymer surfaces was also investigated since the ionically bonded heparin could dissociate from the quaternary ammonium groups at the surface. Indeed, as will be discussed later, ionically bonded heparin does, in fact, slowly dissociate from the surface in the presence of blood. The heparin molecule has carboxylic acid, hydroxyl, and amino groups available for covalent attachment. A number of different reagents and heparin derivatives were employed [4] such as the acid hydrazide of heparin, silylated heparin, an ethyleneimine-heparin derivative, a carbodiimide-heparin derivative, and a heparin-cyanuric chloride adduct. Of these, the best results in terms of the amounts of heparin bound were achieved with the cyanuric chloride adduct. Heparin was first reacted with cyanuric chloride to form a derivative which had approximately seven

residues per heparin molecule (based on a molecular weight of
15,000) and which retained 85 percent of its anticoagulant activity.
Attachment to silicone rubber was effected through first bonding
the amino groups to the silicone rubber by means of aminopropyltriethoxysilane followed by reaction with the heparin derivative.
This method resulted in large amounts of bound heparin (50-
100 μg/sq cm) which could not be displaced by 4N sodium chloride
solutions. The fact that the heparin linked via cyanuric chloride
could not be displaced with salt indicated covalent bonding since
ionically bonded heparin is almost completely displaced under
similar conditions. Surprisingly enough, surfaces containing covalently bonded heparin did not perform well when implanted in
animals. Possible reasons for this will be discussed in a later
section.

All of the above methods for surface attachment of heparin
required chemical modification of the surface. Thus, heparinization by many of these processes could often be time consuming
and, in some cases, could result in damage to the surface, such
as crazing, roughness, or opacification. In addition, most of the
processes were specific for a given material. In order to heparinize a composite device, a separate process for each different
material in the device would be required. For these reasons,
after the general efficacy of heparinized surfaces had been established, further work on heparinization was directed toward the
development of rapid and broadly applicable methods. Since covalent attachment reactions are specific for given polymers, heparinization via adsorption of the quaternary ammonium compound
was explored. Quaternary ammonium salts containing a single
long chain alkyl are easily displaced from polymer surfaces and
thus would not be acceptable. However, quaternary ammonium
salts with three long alkyl groups are water insoluble and are not
easily displaced from a surface in contact with an aqueous phase.
For this reason, tridodecylmethylammonium chloride (TDMAC)
was investigated as a means of attaching heparin to a large number
of polymers by a broadly applicable and simple technique. In the
original work, a solution of TDMAC in an organic solvent was used
as a first step in this process. The material was simply dipped
in this solution, dried, and then exposed to an 0.25 percent solution
of heparin in water. The method proved to be generally applicable
for a large number of different polymers [5] and resulted in the
attachment of large amounts of heparin as shown in Table I.

TABLE I

ATTACHMENT OF HEPARIN TO POLYMERS WITH TDMAC

Polymer	Amount of Heparin on Surface, µg/sq cm		
	Initial	Percent after 100 hrs in saline	Percent after 4 hrs in plasma
Polyvinyl chloride	25	100	95
Polycarbonate	4	93	90
Mylar	18	95	90
Silicone rubber	22	91	-
Polyurethane	186	100	98
Polyethylene	25	100	94
Polypropylene	8.2	92	91
Teflon	1.1	99	87

Measured as S^{35}-labeled heparin

As can be seen from the table, the heparin attached to the surface was quite stable and very little was removed after four hours contact with blood plasma. This technique had the advantage over previous methods of heparinization in its simplicity and speed and also because it enabled the treatment of composite devices containing several different polymers. Thus, an artificial heart device constructed from silicone rubber, polypropylene, and polycarbonate could be heparinized in one simple procedure.

Further improvement has been made on the TDMAC process by the development of the one-step treatment [6]. This technique takes advantage of the ability of heparin to form an organic soluble complex with TDMAC at appropriate ratios of heparin to the quaternary ammonium salt. To make the complex, an aqueous solution of heparin is briefly shaken with a toluene solution of TDMAC during which time the complex forms and dissolves in the toluene. This complex can then be utilized to heparinize polymers in a simple one-step process which consists of dipping the material for a short time into a one percent solution of the complex followed by air drying. The length of time of exposure varies according to the polymer but for most materials is only a few seconds. The resulting surfaces are stable and can be sterilized by either autoclaving or ethylene oxide.

Several other investigators [7, 8, 9, 10, 11, 12, 13] have developed heparinized surfaces in which heparin is attached either by covalent or ionic bonding. Several different substrate materials have been utilized including cellophane, silicone rubber, and polyethylene. In general, these materials have greatly improved non-thrombogenicity. A detailed discussion of each of these materials is beyond the scope of this paper.

CHARACTERISTICS OF HEPARINIZED SURFACES

The interactions of heparinized surfaces with blood have been evaluated by a number of in vivo, ex vivo, and in vitro systems. When whole blood is placed in a test tube containing a heparinized surface, it does not clot; however, if the blood is then poured into a glass tube, clotting occurs within five minutes. This shows that the heparinized surface does not work by simply anticoagulating the blood. Ex vivo experiments by other investigators [14] have shown the TDMAC-heparinized surfaces to be the most thrombo-resistant of all materials investigated thus far. In these experiments, blood was passed directly from a dog into a chamber coated with test materials in which a vortex was generated. The vortex stimulated clot formation and the amount of clot was influenced by the type of surface.

The thrombogenicity of these surfaces has been evaluated by numerous animal studies. In one of the studies, TDMAC-heparinized rings were implanted in the venae cavae of dogs and were found completely free of clots [15] in marked contrast to control surfaces which were completely occluded. In other studies, these surfaces were used successfully in membrane oxygenation in the absence of systemic heparinization [16] and in indwelling vascular cannulae [17].

The TDMAC-heparinized surfaces now are undergoing clinical studies by a large number of investigators. Our laboratories are currently preparing heparinized devices of many different configurations. The device with the largest number of clinical trials to date is a shunt used in the repair of thoracic aneurysms [18, 19]. In this technique, a treated polyvinyl chloride shunt is used without systemic heparinization to divert the blood from the aorta to

the femoral artery while the aorta is repaired. We have prepared
over 700 of these shunts and sent them to 130 clinical investigators.
The TDMAC-heparin process has also been successfully used with
heart valves in humans. In addition, we have heparinized over 100
shunts for repair of carotid aneurysms and numerous types of cannulae used for access to the cardiovascular system. The results
from these studies indicate that the heparinized surfaces have very
low thrombogenicity in contact with blood.

The mechanism by which heparinized surfaces are nonthrombogenic is not well understood at the present time. When heparinized
surfaces are placed in contact with blood, adsorption of proteins
occurs very rapidly. The pattern of adsorption of the major plasma
proteins by heparinized surfaces does not seem to vary significantly
from that of the underlying polymer [20]. The adsorption and interaction of these surfaces with the components of the coagulation
system has not been studied in detail. Our work, as well as work
by Salzman, et al. [21], indicates that heparinized surfaces do not
activate the Hageman factor, a protein which is involved in the initiation of surface-induced coagulation.

Another characteristic of most surfaces containing ionically
bound heparin is the elution of small amounts of heparin when the
surfaces are contacted with blood. As mentioned previously, blood
placed in a heparinized test tube clots normally and thus normal
anticoagulation does not occur. In studies with radiolabeled heparin [22], workers in our laboratory showed that heparin was released in small amounts from particulated heparinized materials
placed in a column in contact with plasma. The rate of release
was high initially and then diminished to a very low level within
two hours after contact. Heparinized carotid-jugular shunts implanted in rabbits had 25 percent of the original heparin remaining
after one week [5]. The shunts were patent in spite of the loss of
heparin.

Another characteristic of heparinized surfaces observed by us
[5] and other workers [23] is the adhesion of platelets. In in vitro
experiments using a column packed with heparin attached to small
(200 μ) particles of silicone rubber, we found that most of the
platelets were removed from the initial fractions of platelet-rich
plasma eluted through the column. Equilibrium was quickly established, however, and subsequent fractions did not have platelets
removed. Similarly, the surfaces of heparinized materials implanted in animals were covered with platelets even though no

thrombus formed. Results of several studies both in our laboratory and by Salzman, et al. have indicated that although platelet
adhesion does occur on heparinized surfaces, subsequent platelet
metamorphosis and release of intracellular constituents does not
occur. Evidently, a relatively benign layer of platelets is deposited on the surface and this layer is not involved in further thrombogenesis.

Recent work has shown that heparinized surfaces bind heparin
cofactor [23, 24]. This binding is quite strong and occurs in the
presence of other plasma proteins. The adsorbed heparin cofactor
is capable of neutralizing thrombin and this may explain in part the
nonthrombogenic properties of heparinized surfaces.

As stated previously, the mechanism by which heparinized
surfaces act is not well understood. They do not act by releasing
large amounts sufficient to anticoagulate the blood. Yet, the fact
that covalently bound heparin surfaces do not perform nearly as
well as those containing ionically bound heparin, implies that heparin must have a certain degree of mobility at the surface. At present, the most attractive hypothesis to explain the mechanism is
that small amounts of heparin are released in the microenviron-
ment of the surface and that this released heparin can effectively
block thrombogenesis at the surface. The presence of heparin at
the surface may also determine the nature of the adsorbed protein
layer and cause the deposition of a benign layer. Thus, the surface remains free of clots long after the initially bound heparin is
gone.

In summary, heparin can be attached to many different polymers by means of a TDMAC complex. The resulting surfaces
have a marked reduction in thrombogenicity and are now finding
practical use in clinical applications.

REFERENCES

1.   Gott, V. L., Whiffen, J. D., and Dutton, R. C., Science,
     142, 1297 (1963).

2.   Leininger, R. I., Cooper, C. W., Epstein, M. M., Falb,
     R. D., and Grode, G. A., ibid., 152, 1625 (1966).

3.   Falb, R. D., Grode, G. A., Luttinger, M., Epstein, M. M.,
     Drake, B., and Leininger, R. I., Development of Blood-
     Compatible Polymeric Materials, U. S. Nat. Tech. Inform.
     Serv., PB Rept. No. 173,053, 1966.

4.   Falb, R. D., Grode, G. A., Grotta, H. M., Wright, R. A.,
     Poirier, R. H., Takahashi, M. T., and Leininger, R. I.,
     Development of Blood-Compatible Materials, U. S. Nat.
     Tech. Inform. Serv., PB Rept. Nos. 175,668, 1967; 183,317,
     1967; 188,108, 1968; and 188,111, 1969.

5.   Grode, G. A., et al., Biocompatible Materials for Use in
     the Vascular System, U. S. Nat. Tech. Inform. Serv.,
     PB Rept. Nos. 188,108, 1969; 195,727, 1970; and 205,475,
     1971.

6.   Leininger, R. I., Falb, R. D., Crowley, J. P., and Grode,
     G. A., Trans. Amer. Soc. Artif. Intern. Organs, 18, 312
     (1972).

7.   Eriksson, J. C., Gillberg, G., and Lagergren, H.,
     J. Biomed. Mater. Res., 1, 301 (1967).

8.   Lagergren, H. and Eriksson, J. C., Trans. Amer. Soc.
     Artif. Intern. Organs, 17, 10 (1971).

9.   Merrill, E. W., Salzman, E. W., Lipps, B. J., Jr.,
     Gilliland, E. R., Austen, W. G., and Joison, J., ibid.,
     12, 139 (1966).

10. Salzman, E. W., Austen, W. G., Lipps, B. J., Jr.,
     Merrill, E. W., and Joison, J., Surgery, 61, 1 (1967).

11. Merrill, E. W., Salzman, E. W., Wong, P.S.L., and
     Ashford, T. P., J. Appl. Physiol., 29, 723 (1970).

12. Halpern, B. D. and Shibakawa, R., in Interactions of Liquids
     at Solid Substrates, R. F. Gould, Ed., American Chemical
     Society, 1968.

13. Merker, R. L., Elyash, L. J., Mayhew, S. H., and Wang,
     J.Y.C., in Proceedings of the Artificial Heart Program
     Conference, R. J. Hegyeli, Ed., National Heart Institute
     Artificial Heart Program, Washington, D.C., 1969, p. 29.

14. Leonard, E. F., in Proceedings of the 5th Annual Contractors' Conference of the Artificial Kidney Program of the National Institute of Arthritis and Metabolic Diseases, K. K. Krueger, Ed., Bethesda, Md., 1972, p. 184.

15. Gott, V. L., Ramos, M. D., Najjar, F. B., Allen, J. L., and Becker, K. E., in Proceedings of the Artificial Heart Program Conference, R. J. Hegyeli, Ed., National Heart Institute Artificial Heart Program, Washington, D.C., 1969, p. 181.

16. Rea, W. J., Whitley, D., and Eberle, J. W., Trans. Amer. Soc. Artif. Intern. Organs, 18, 316 (1972).

17. Kowarski, A., Thompson, R. G., Migeon, C. J., and Blizzard, R. M., J. Clin. Endocrinol., 30, 356 (1971).

18. Krause, A. H., Ferguson, T. B., and Weldon, C. S., Ann. Thorac. Surg., 14, 123 (1972).

19. Brenner, W. I., Engelman, R. M., Williams, C. D., Boyd, A. D., and Reed, G. E., Amer. J. Surg., 127, 555 (1974).

20. Mobin-Uddin, K., Utley, J. R., Bryant, L. R., Dillon, M., and Weiss, D. L., Ann. Thorac. Surg., 17, 351 (1974).

21. Salzman, E. W., Merrill, E. G., Binder, A., Wolf, C.F.W., Ashford, T. P., and Austen, W. G., J. Biomed. Mater. Res., 3, 69 (1969).

22. Falb, R. D., Takahashi, M. T., Grode, G. A., and Leininger, R. I., ibid., 1, 239 (1967).

23. Gentry, P. and Alexander, B., Biochem. Biophys. Res. Commun., 50, 500 (1973).

24. Thaler, E. and Schmer, G., Abstracts, 20th Annual Meeting of the American Society for Artificial Internal Organs, Chicago, Ill., April 3-5, 1974, p. 73.

SILICONES

John W. Boretos

Biomedical Engineering and Instrumentation Branch,
Division of Research Sciences, National Institutes of
Health, Bethesda, Maryland 20012

INTRODUCTION

Marked acceleration in the development of surrogate surgical
implants has taken place over the past 20 years. As a direct consequence, previously intractable difficulties such as hydrocephalus,
heart-block, incompetent heart valves and others are now being
challenged successfully. All of these are dependent upon inert
materials, in some form, for safe and efficacious performance.
Fortuitously, the introduction of silicones in pure form coincided
with this demand.

Although the advantages of silicones were first recognized in
the food processing industry, it was elastomeric baby-bottle nipples and nonwetting silicone coatings for glass that called these
materials to the attention of biomedical researchers. The nipples
were safe for babies to chew and did not deteriorate with repeated
sterilizing; the clotting time of blood in vitro was extended by a
coating of silicone on contact surfaces. Today, major "standard"
implants and many custom-made devices are made from silicone
rubber because very few substitutes perform as well in the very
demanding environment within the human body. Literally hundreds
of thousands of patients have benefited.

Despite this impressive record, it must be realized that no
single material is perfect for all situations. Successful performance depends upon the judicious selection of not only the proper

structure and properties of substances but upon the manner and
environment in which they are to be used. Simple prescriptions
for compatibility cannot be devised where the inanimate must
function in place of or in proximity to living tissues. Each application must be selectively tailored on the basis of past experience
with similar devices in like circumstances. The purpose of this
paper is to describe the structure and function of medically useful
silicones, their limitations and their attributes.

CHEMICAL DESCRIPTION

Numerous silicone rubber products are regularly used in industry; many of these, however, are unsuitable for use in the body
because of toxic catalysts, fillers, or additives. Medically approved silicones, although they may possess various components,
must be innocuous.

The basic structure of the medical silicones consists, essentially, of repeating linear chains of dimethyl siloxane polymers as
described in detail, for example, by Braley [1]. They are produced by converting silica to silicon which is then treated with
methyl chloride to form dimethyl dichlorosilane. The latter reacts
with water to form an unstable diol which spontaneously condenses
to form a silicone polymer terminated by hydroxyl groups. These
are converted, with the controlled addition of hexamethyl disiloxane,
to form the methyl terminated siloxane polymer gum:

$$\left[-\underset{\underset{CH_3}{|}}{\overset{\overset{CH_3}{|}}{Si}} - O - \right]_n$$

polysiloxane

The gum, a water-white, clear, highly viscous fluid, is the basic
form from which the various types of silicone elastomers developed.
Table I outlines the typical medical silicones. Much of the inertness of the polymer compared to natural rubber, for example, is
thought to originate in the strength of the silicone-oxygen bond
(i.e., 108 Kcal for Si-O versus 83 Kcal for C-C bonds).

TABLE I

TYPICAL TYPES OF MEDICAL SILICONES

---

1. Heat Vulcanizing
   A. Firm
   B. Medium
   C. Soft
   D. Others
      Fluorosilicone
      Polycarbonate/silicone copolymer

2. Room Temperature Vulcanizing
   A. One component system
   B. Two component system

3. Fluids

Heat Vulcanizing Silicone

Heat vulcanizing silicone rubber, which offers the greatest degree of strength of all available silicone compounds, has been used most often for fabricating implants. This polymer, composed of dimethyl siloxane, can have additional groups such as methyl vinyl siloxane and/or phenylmethyl siloxane dispersed throughout its chains. The purpose of the vinyl groups is to enhance crosslinking and suitability for use with general purpose catalysts. This form is preferred for heart valve poppets and medical tubing. The phenyl groups provide for a softer form of rubber and low-temperature resistance. In the presence of a crosslinking agent, the vinyl group of one chain is united with the methyl group of another chain to achieve the crosslinked state. For a more chemically resistant grade of silicone, the basic structure previously described can have fluorine functional groups attached to the siloxy unit; an example is 3,3,3-trifluoropropyl-methyl siloxane. Work by Musolf and associates [2] suggests that this type of silicone rubber is more thromboresistant than others. Combined with its improved oil resistance, which could indicate low lipid solubility, this material may prove advantageous for heart valve poppets to counter deterioration due to lipid adsorption from the blood.

Type I

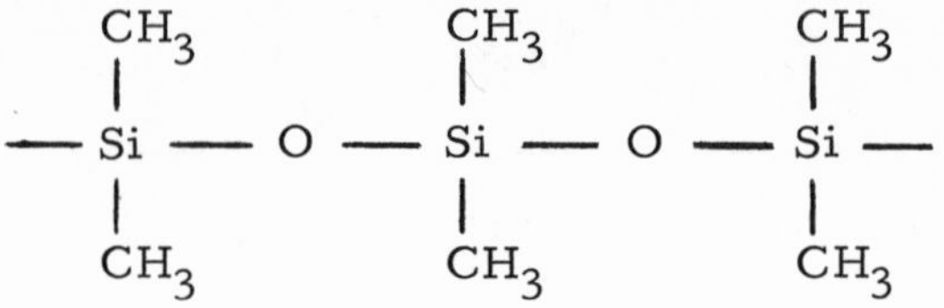

$$\begin{array}{ccccc} & CH_3 & & CH_3 & & CH_3 \\ & | & & | & & | \\ -\!\!\!-Si\!\!-\!\!O\!\!-\!\!Si\!\!-\!\!O\!\!-\!\!Si\!\!-\!\! \\ & | & & | & & | \\ & CH_3 & & CH_3 & & CH_3 \end{array}$$

Type II

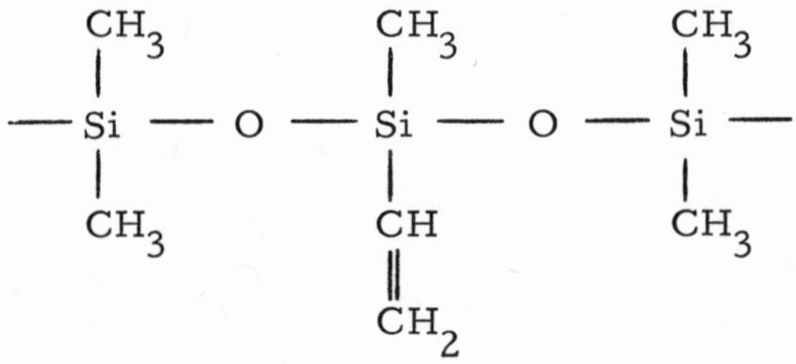

$$\begin{array}{ccccc} & CH_3 & & CH_3 & & CH_3 \\ & | & & | & & | \\ -\!\!\!-Si\!\!-\!\!O\!\!-\!\!Si\!\!-\!\!O\!\!-\!\!Si\!\!-\!\! \\ & | & & | & & | \\ & CH_3 & & CH & & CH_3 \\ & & & \| \\ & & & CH_2 \end{array}$$

Type III

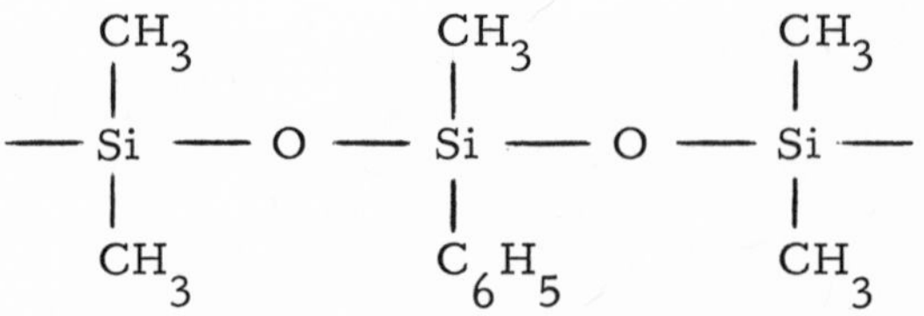

$$\begin{array}{ccccc} & CH_3 & & CH_3 & & CH_3 \\ & | & & | & & | \\ -\!\!\!-Si\!\!-\!\!O\!\!-\!\!Si\!\!-\!\!O\!\!-\!\!Si\!\!-\!\! \\ & | & & | & & | \\ & CH_3 & & C_6H_5 & & CH_3 \end{array}$$

Type IV

$$\begin{array}{ccccc} & CH_3 & & CH_3 & & CH_3 \\ & | & & | & & | \\ -\!\!\!-Si\!\!-\!\!O\!\!-\!\!Si\!\!-\!\!O\!\!-\!\!Si\!\!-\!\! \\ & | & & | & & | \\ & CH_3 & & CH_2 & & CH_3 \\ & & & | \\ & & & CH_2 \\ & & & | \\ & & & CF_3 \end{array}$$

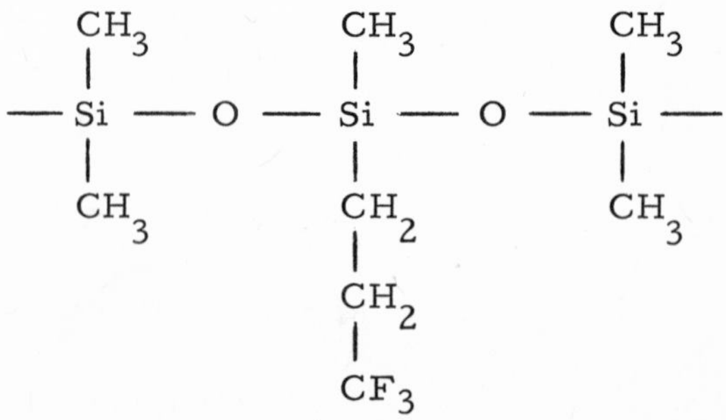

FIGURE 1. Typical structures of the medical grade silicone gums.

TABLE II

OXYGEN AND CARBON DIOXIDE PERMEABILITY OF DIMETHYL SILOXANE VS SILICONE POLY- CARBONATE COPOLYMER [3]

Material	Permeability* O_2	CO_2
Dimethyl siloxane	50	270
Silicone/polycarbonate copolymer	16	97

$$* \left[10^{-9} \ \frac{\text{cc gas (RTP) cm}}{\text{sec, sq cm, cm Hg } \Delta P} \right]$$

Figure 1 shows the four main types of silicone gum from which crosslinked medical elastomers are made. There are generally about 5000 to 9000 of these units in each polymer chain. Type I is polydimethyl siloxane. Type II is essentially Type I with a small fraction of methyl groups replaced by vinyl groups. Type III has phenyl groups replacing some methyl groups and Type IV is trifluoropropylmethyl siloxane with a small level of methylvinyl siloxane included (not indicated in figure).

Silicones are well known for their high degree of gas permeability, especially to carbon dioxide and oxygen, an asset for use in artificial oxygenators. Combining polycarbonate and silicone in the form of a copolymer, retains permeability and adds significantly to the overall strength and tear resistance of thin films and capillaries. Table II shows the gas permeability of dimethyl siloxane compared with that of the silicone/polycarbonate copolymer. Knazek and co-workers [4] have used this material for providing O_2, along with other capillaries permeable to nutrients, to good advantage in producing a viable environment for propagating cancer cells in vitro.

Room Temperature Vulcanizing Silicones

Room temperature vulcanizing (RTV) silicone compounds are liquids and pastes that cure to solid, resilient elastomers suitable for medical use. They can be divided into two groups: (a) the single component system and (b) the two component system. The former is exemplified by the popular adhesives commercially available in squeeze-tube form. Here hydroxyl-terminated methyl siloxane is present with methyl triacetoxysilane. When the mixture is exposed to moisture from the air, the acetoxy groups are cleaved from the methyl triacetoxysilane and transformed into volatile acetic acid and methylsilane having multiple hydroxyl groups. The latter spontaneously combines with the hydroxyl-terminated methylsilane present to extend the polymer chain and to form suitable crosslinks. Raw silicone rubber readily bonds to other silicones and offers a conveninet means for fabricating seams of pacemakers, artificial hearts, and numerous other applications. The two component system is best known as a potting or encapsulating compound. Here hydroxyl-terminated methylsilane is packaged in combination with propylorthosilicate as one component. With the additon of the second component, the catalyst, the hydroxyl groups react to split off the alkyl groups and polymer is then available to crosslink through the remaining silicate. These RTVs have been used to encapsulate implantable electronic pacemakers and telemetry devices, insulate indwelling electrodes, and to form molds for fabricating artificial heart valves and other components. Because they can be readily tinted, they have also been used to cosmetically reconstruct maxillofacial deformities.

Fluids

Silicone fluids are similar to the elastomers differing only in viscosity, molecular weight and potential for crosslinking. Medical silicone fluid has been classified as "a new drug use" by the Food and Drug Administration; its sale is controlled by law. Regulations are deemed necessary to prevent indiscriminate use of the material for tissue augmentation, especially in the breast where migration and scarring have resulted from inappropriate use. Under the proper conditions, using tiny droplets well dispersed throughout the tissues, silicone fluids exhibit minimal loss from the injection site [5] and no adverse tissue reaction. These same fluids, however, can be detrimental when applied to the delicate

TABLE III

TYPICAL PHYSICAL PROPERTIES OF MEDICAL SILICONE ELASTOMERS

Type	Property			Description
	Tensile strength psi	Elongation %	Hardness Shore A	
Heat vulcanizing				
a. Firm	1000	350	75	MDX 4-4516 (raw form), Silastic 373 (vulcan. form), Dow Corning Corp.
b. Medium	1200	450	50	MDX 4-4515 (raw form), Silastic 372 (vulcan. form), Dow Corning Corp.
c. Soft	850	600	25	MDX 4-4514 (raw form), Silastic 370 (vulcan. form), Dow Corning Corp.
d. Fluorosilicone	1000	250	55	MDX 4-4026
e. Silicone/polycarbonate	2600	-	-	MEM 213, GE Co. Autoclave at 250°F, heat sealable, thermoplastic, less permeable to $O_2 + CO_2$ than A, B, C, D but durable in thin sections.
One component RTV	300	450	28	Adhesive A, Dow Corning Corp., clear.
Two component RTV	400	160	43	Silastic 382, Dow Corning Corp., white potting compound.
	700	420	32	MDX 4-4210, Dow Corning Corp., clear potting compound.

tissues of the eye. Contact, over an extended period, with the iris, cornea, or lens can cause scarring, vascularization, edema, and atrophy.

PROPERTIES

Physical Properties

Reinforcing agents are necessary in silicone rubber formulations to provide strength and bulk. For example, the tensile strength of a vulcanized gum can be increased from 100 psi to over 1000 psi with proper compounding. Fine particle silicas are the most effective reinforcing agents for heat vulcanizing stocks and produce rubber that is strong and "snappy" with high elongations. Diatomaceous earths are preferred for the RTV potting compounds because they possess the best balance of handling properties and strength for these liquid systems. To add radiopaque qualities to silicone rubber, barium sulfate can be safely milled into the various types and has been used in heart valve poppets and catheters to enable movement visualization. Table III summarizes the physical properties of the most commonly used medical silicone elastomers.

Stability

Swanson and Le Beau [6] have studied the change in physical properties of heat vulcanized silicone rubber implanted subcutaneously in beagle dogs. They concluded that slight changes do occur which should not alter material performance. A maximum gain in weight of 0.91% was observed which stabilized in about four weeks; gain was due mainly to lipid absorption. They further determined that although extractable silicone polymer was present in the test specimen, it did not leach into the body or influence lipid uptake or physical properties. Table IV summarizes their findings. Developers of artificial heart valves have relied heavily upon silicone rubber for many designs. The ball-in-cage variety has been implanted in an estimated 25,000 patients. A small percentage of these, most in the aortic position, have been adversely affected by blood "lipids" requiring replacement. Carmen and Kahn [7] have shown that in vitro lipid absorption increased with degree of cure and decreased with silica filler content. They found the "lipid" to consist of fatty acids, neutral fat, steroid,

TABLE IV

STABILITY OF MEDICAL SILICONE RUBBER
IMPLANTED IN DOGS* [6]

Property	Value for control	Percent change		
		4 wks	6 mos	2 yrs
Tensile strength	1388 psi	-	- 7	- 8
Ultimate elongation	377 %	-	-10	-15
Modulus @ 200%	506 psi	-	+ 8	+16
Weight**	-	+0.75	+ 0.91	+ 0.63

*Based on two beagle dogs.
**Attributed to lipid absorption; generally stable after four wks.

steroid ester, and phospholipid and was present from 0.1 to
5.5 wt % when associated with 4% increase by volume. Eight hours
at lowered post-curing temperatures (i.e. 250°F) was found to reduce the lipid uptake (0.82 wt %). In vivo improvement as a result
of this scheme has been indicated but is not conclusively documented.

Biocompatibility

The common use of additives to achieve specific properties
in most industrial elastomers of outstanding chemical resistance
such as trifluorochloroethylene, polychloroprene, vinylidene
fluoride/hexafluoropropylene copolymer, is precluded by the potential adverse effects of eluting components. In tailoring silicones
for medical use, the approach has been to minimize complications
by keeping the system as simple and inert as possible. Crosslinking agents must be chosen carefully since they significantly
influence the properties of the finished rubber. For the heat vulcanizing systems, several organic peroxides can be used.
2,4-Dichlorobenzoyl peroxide is often used with medical grade
stocks because of its molding versatility. A small amount is dispersed during compounding and, when the rubber is heated above
a critical temperature, the peroxide decomposes to an active free

radical to induce crosslinking; the agent and breakdown products can be driven off with further heating. For the RTV two component system, stannous octoate is the least toxic of those commonly used. Here it is especially important to select a nontoxic material because this crosslinking agent is a true catalyst which remains in the vulcanized rubber as an uncombined entity. Thorough mixing is required to insure even distribution throughout the mass for consistent results.

Silicone has the ability to retard the clotting of blood when applied to active surfaces such as glass. For this reason it is widely used in devices for withdrawing blood test samples. The thromboresistance that silicone rubber exhibits in vivo depends directly upon details of technique and circumstance. For example, a vessel replacement made of silicone in a low flow area will most likely clot, whereas a silicone rubber catheter placed within the same area can function effectively, depending upon how much foreign surface is exposed, flow patterns, surface characteristics and geometry. In high flow areas or in larger vessels, both devices may stimulate only minimal emboli or clots that can be carried away or lysed before a significant mass can develop. Arterio-venous shunts for kidney dialysis and hydrocephalus valves are examples. This type of performance is difficult to predict because of incomplete knowledge of the clotting events. Nyilas [8] suggests that minor formulation variables and the presence of silica-rich areas in silicone rubber can adversely influence the clotting mechanism. Numerous investigators have attempted to permanently bond heparin to silicone surfaces to obtain enduring thromboresistance. A completely desirable system has not yet been devised.

DISCUSSION

The hydrocephalus valve is, perhaps, the most extensively used silicone implant device. Since its introduction in 1955, over 150,000 patients have received them [5] to alleviate cerebral fluid pressure buildup. The valve consists of a short length of tubing, with an internal slit, that extends between the ventricle of the brain and the right auricle of the heart. Variations include automatic flushing via an in-line reservoir chamber or direct drain into the peritoneal cavity. Thousands of silicone rubber bands have been placed permanently around the eye as part of a surgical procedure to repair detached retinas. Mammary augmentation has been performed extensively using silicone rubber bags filled with either a

pure form of silicone gel or filled with an isotonic fluid after implantation. Thousands of finger and toe joints destroyed by arthritis are being replaced by hinge-like silicone prostheses. Some
failures have been associated with accidental cuts or improper
alignment. Although carpal, radial, and ulnar heads have been
replaced, major joint supplantation is not possible because silicone
rubber lacks the required load-bearing strength.

The number of useful medical devices produced from silicone
rubber is enormous and increasing steadily. Representative lists
have been published [9, 10]. Specific applications have been mentioned here solely for the purpose of illustrating capabilities and
calling attention to typical limitations of this most useful class of
polymers. Many have been misled into frustration and failure because of the apparently simple nature of the silicone elastomers.
It cannot be overemphasized that extremely careful attention to
detail in formulation, design, and application is critical if the
potential of this unique life preserving polymer is to be realized.

SUMMARY

Medical silicones have proven invaluable for numerous surgical implants. Although the heat vulcanizing types are generally
regarded as the most durable, the room temperature vulcanizing
varieties can serve invaluable functions in many critical applications as well. The ability of silicone rubber to resist mechanical
stresses is limited and must be considered carefully in designing
for dynamic or load-bearing applications. Although a number of
prostheses have functioned well in the vascular system, adverse
phenomena such as clotting and physical and chemical changes
can occur depending upon circumstances. Each application must
be tailored specifically and carefully if success is to be achieved.

REFERENCES

1. Braley, S., J. Macromol. Sci.-Chem., A4, 529 (1970).

2. Musolf, M. C., Hulce, V. D., Bennett, D. R., and Ramos,
    M., Trans. Amer. Soc. Artif. Intern. Organs, 15, 18 (1969).

3. General Electric Permaselective Membranes, Data Sheet,
    General Electric Co, Schenectady, N. Y.

4. Knazek, R. A., Gullino, P. M., Kohler, P. O., and Dedrick,
    R. L., Science, 178, 65 (1972).

5. Braley, S. A., in Modern Trends in Biomechanics, D. C.
    Simpson, Ed., Appleton-Century-Crofts, New York, 1970.

6. Swanson, J. W. and Le Beau, J. E., The Effect of Implan-
    tation on the Physical Properties of Silicone Rubber. Un-
    published data.

7. Carmen, R. and Kahn, P., J. Biomed. Mater. Res. 2, 457
    (1968).

8. Nyilas, E., Kupski, E. L., Burnett, P., and Haag, R. M.,
    ibid., 4, 371 (1970).

9. Lee, H. and Neville, K., Handbook of Biomedical Plastics,
    Pasadena Technology Press, Pasadena, Calif., 1971.

10. Boretos, J. W., Concise Guide to Biomedical Polymers:
    Their Design, Fabrication, and Molding, Charles C. Thomas,
    Springfield, Ill., 1973.

MEMBRANES

Harold B. Hopfenberg

Department of Chemical Engineering, North Carolina
State University, Raleigh, North Carolina 27607

BRIEF RECENT HISTORY OF MEMBRANE SEPARATIONS

As recently as 15 years ago, membrane separations were considered primarily for the separation and purification of organic mixtures. Typical applications were specialty isomer separations and the separation of organic liquids with very similar volatilities [1].

The development of highly selective and relatively high through-put membranes for aqueous separations prompted a marked shift in the emphasis of the research and development toward high volume, commonly encountered separations such as desalination, demineralization, and by-product recovery. Moreover, these advances in membrane technology for aqueous systems made membrane separation attractive for a variety of medically-related separations.

Much of the membrane-related research of the 1960s was directed toward modifying membrane materials and toward the development of novel membrane configurations. Although cellulose and cellulose acetate membranes formed the keystone of this emerging research, hundreds of candidate polymers were screened for potential application as selective barriers for a variety of aqueous separations [2]. In general, these studies attempted to correlate polymer structure with product flux and solute retention of the membrane material. Strikingly imaginative developments led

to the asymmetric, high flux membrane [3] and the hollow fine
fiber which provides exceedingly high membrane area per unit
equipment volume [4]. Throughout this period, studies of gas
permeation of polymer membranes were pursued. These studies
were motivated by the requirements for improved barrier materials for packaging as well as the continuing search for semiper-
meable membranes to effect gas separations [5].

LIMITING TRANSPORT MECHANISMS: SOLUTION-DIFFUSION MODEL VS PORE FLOW

There are two limiting mechanisms governing the transport
of small molecules in and through selective membranes. In fact,
many separations are effected by truly consolidated membranes.
In this case, the only available mechanism for transport is activated diffusion involving the cooperative motion of polymeric moieties or segments and the diffusing penetrant. This mechanism,
termed the solution-diffusion model, is described simply for a
given component by the following expression:

$$\overline{P} = Dk$$

where $\overline{P}$ is a steady state permeability, D is a diffusion coefficient,
and k is an equilibrium solubility. The permeability, therefore,
is the simple product of diffusivity (which may be considered as a
kinetic parameter) and a solubility (which is a thermodynamic
parameter). Although molecular size and shape of the diffusing
species affects the diffusion coefficient and, in turn, the permeability in a regular, predictable, and understandable manner the
equilibrium solubility is determined by much more complex and
seemingly abstract considerations. In fact, solubilities generally
increase with increasing molecular size which makes simple predictions of steady state permeabilities, on the basis of size and
shape alone, rather difficult.

Penetrants that dissolve only sparingly (low k) will permeate
a membrane relatively slowly, whereas large molecules, with
predictably low values of D, will similarly permeate slowly.
Simply, considerations of size and shape tell only half the story
for a "solution-diffusion" membrane.

TABLE I

THE PERMEABILITY OF VARIOUS POLYMERS TO OXYGEN WATER AND CARBON DIOXIDE AT 30°C

Material	P_{O_2}	P_{CO_2}	Ratio P_{CO_2}/P_{O_2}	P_{H_2O}
Polyacrylonitrile	0.0002	0.0008	4.0	300
Polymethacrylonitrile	0.0012	0.0032	2.7	410
Lopac (Monsanto Co.)*	0.0035	0.0108	3.1	340
Polyvinylidene chloride	0.0053	0.029	5.5	1.0
Barex (Sohio Co.)*	0.0054	0.061	3.4	660
Polyethylene terephthalate	0.035	0.017	4.9	175
Nylon 6	0.038	0.016	3.6	275
Polyvinyl chloride (unplast.)	0.045	0.016	3.6	275
Polyethylene (dens. 0.964)	0.40	1.80	4.5	12
Cellulose acetate (unplast.)	0.080	2.40	3.0	6,800
Butyl rubber	1.30	5.18	4.0	120
Polycarbonate	1.40	8.0	5.7	1,400
Polypropylene (dens. 0.907)	2.20	9.2	4.2	65
Polystyrene	2.63	10.5	3.8	1,200
Polyethylene (dens. 0.922)	6.90	28.0	4.0	90
Neoprene	4.0	25.8	6.5	910
Teflon	4.9	12.7	2.6	33.0
Poly(2,6-dimethyl 1,4-phenylene oxide)	15.8	75.7	4.8	4,060
Natural rubber	23.3	153	6.6	2,600
Poly(4-methyl pentene-1)	32.3	92.6	2.9	-
Polydimethyl siloxane	605	3,240	5.3	40,000

*Nitrile copolymers
Units: CCS. (S.T.P.)/sq cm/cm/sec/cm Hg x 10^{10}

The large compilation of data presented in Table I* indicates that the larger CO_2 molecule exhibits higher permeabilities through a variety of polymer films. This increased permeability is a manifestation of the higher solubility of CO_2 in these various polymers.

Alternatively, polymeric membranes can be produced with controlled porosity. These membranes indeed exclude dissolved molecular species on the basis of size and shape alone, quite analagous to conventional filters which separate suspended material from two phase suspensions and slurries. The commonly used terms reverse osmosis and ultrafiltration are described in the following section; these terms are defined independent of the specific mechanisms controlling transport. Both processes involve the retention of truly dissolved species by the selective membrane although in either process the membrane may function by a "solution-diffusion" or a "pore-flow" mechanism. In some ultrafiltration processes, very high molecular weight species may be retained while low molecular weight solutes and salts are freely transported with the carrier solvent across the membrane. Although related, this process should not be confused with solute dialysis which operates strictly on the basis of a concentration gradient of solute in the absence of a hydrostatic pressure gradient.

ULTRAFILTRATION AND REVERSE OSMOSIS

The field of pressure driven membrane separations has become so broad that it is convenient and useful to divide these membrane separations into two major categories termed reverse osmosis and ultrafiltration. Reverse osmosis describes membrane separations involving solute concentrations sufficiently high to generate osmotic pressures which are significant when compared with the operating pressure of the process. Ultrafiltration processes operate under virtually identical conditions; the one seemingly small, but exceedingly significant difference is that the molar concentration of solute is sufficiently low so that the osmotic pressure deriving from the presence of solute is negligibly small compared with the operating pressure [6].

---

*V. T. Stannett, personal communication.

This subtle difference between the processes leads to significant differences in the attendant technologies. Reverse osmosis is used primarily for the treatment of solutions of low molecular weight, reasonably high concentration solutes. Ultrafiltration is used for the concentration, fractionation, or dewatering of solutions of macromolecules containing exceedingly low molar concentrations of solute due to the high solute molecular weights. The high molecular weights of the solutes insure the existence of a relatively low osmotic pressure gradient so that, unlike reverse osmosis of microsolute-containing solutions, ultrafiltration requires only moderate operating pressures.

The development of high flux, highly retentive membranes ironically created a problem even more vexing than the limitations inherent in the early membranes. Solute accumulation at the upstream membrane surface is an unfortunate consequence of the development of high flux, highly retentive membranes.

This solute accumulation, termed concentration polarization, at best can only be eliminated by reducing the thickness of the upstream boundary layer in the feed stream. This involves high circulation rates or other techniques for introducing agitation [7]. The practical consequence of concentration polarization is actual process performance which is significantly inferior to the product flux-solute retention behavior theoretically achieved with a given membrane [8, 9].

Recent investigations [10, 11, 12, 13] have dealt with the question of whether this phenomenon is primarily physical (pore blockage by large solute molecules), is primarily an effect resulting from solute aggregation or gel formation adjacent to the membrane, or is primarily the result of specific, functional-group-related interactions between solute molecules and the membrane. These studies are probably the most relevant today since the measures needed to reduce or eliminate flux-limiting effects clearly depend on the specific phenomena causing these effects.

DONNAN EFFECTS IN ION SELECTIVE MEMBRANES

When aqueous solutions are forced through membranes under the influence of a hydrostatic pressure gradient, the presence of a membrane-impermeable ion in the pressurized solution can markedly affect the transport of co-ions through the membrane.

These observations have been explained by extending Donnan's [14] arguments for equilibrium systems, satisfying these exclusion criteria, to the steady-state situations characterizing membrane transport [15].

Donnan's powerful argument predicting equilibrium distribution of ionic species across ion selective (ion-excluding) membranes is based simply on the requirements for equality of the chemical potential of dissolved salts on both sides of the membrane and the additional requirements for equality of total positive and negative charges (charge neutrality) on both sides of the membrane.

These somewhat obvious criteria, coupled with exclusion of a particular ion (say x^-) by the membrane, leads to the following equilibrium distribution of co-anions:

$$c_-''/c_-' = \sqrt{1 + c'_x{}^-/c'_-}$$

where   ' refers to the side of the membrane where x^- ions are exclusively present

        '' is the opposite side of the membrane

        c'_x- refers to the concentrations of x^- in the ' side of the membrane

and

        c_- refers to the concentration of co-anions

Clearly, if there is no x^- present in the system, there would be equality of the "co-ion" concentrations on opposing sides of the membrane. As the concentration of excluded x^- is increased the equilibrium distribution of co-ion skews increasingly toward the opposite side of the membrane.

APPLICATION OF TRANSPORT MODELS AND PROCESSES TO MEDICAL AND PHARMACEUTICAL PROBLEMS

The effective use of ultrafiltration as a separation process began and continues in clinical and related laboratories [16].

Since membranes can be selected which do not denature protein fractions, ultrafiltration is ideal for concentration, desalting, dewatering and related processing of sera. Similarly, purification of an ion-dextran complex (removing sodium chloride, glycol, and citric acid) can be efficiently accomplished by ultrafiltration.

Large scale concentration of serum albumin is currently under extensive evaluation. The continuous removal of waste products from fermentation broths is accomplished by ultrafiltration.

Most frequently membrane processes are identified with ex-corporeal artificial organs. Membrane-based blood oxygenators are probably the simplest application of membrane science to medicine. The consolidated membranes transport oxygen and carbon dioxide countercurrently by a "solution-diffusion" mechanism.

Although the human kidney functions by true ultrafiltration, most artificial kidneys function by dialysis in the absence of a pressure gradient. Porter and Nelson [17] have reported on schemes for eliminating uremic toxins by ultrafiltration rather than by conventional dialysis.

Ultrafiltration, using microporous membranes, has also been used to separate the formed elements from blood plasma on either a batch or continuous basis.

One of the newest and most exciting applications of membrane science to advanced therapeutic techniques is the development of membrane-based devices as implants for controlled and sustained drug release to specific organs. Pilocarpine can be released from a lens-like device by a "solution-diffusion" mechanism to control progressive glaucoma. Similar concepts have been applied to the controlled release of progesterone into the uterus to control female fertility. Other membrane-related devices are in develop-ment to release drugs at a constant rate to the gastrointestinal tract.

The skin has been considered as a port of entry for trans-dermal delivery of drugs. A device applied conveniently to the skin by an adhesive can release drug constantly until administra-tion is terminated abruptly by removal of the patch-like device.

Indeed this one area of membrane-based therapeutics is so limitless and exciting that one-fourth of this conference is devoted to this single area of membrane-based therapeutics. It is intriguing that most of this exciting technology is based upon the simplest of transport mechanisms: "solution-diffusion" of an active drug in the absence of a pressure gradient.

SUMMARY

A brief history of the rapidly developing field of membrane-based separations for gases, vapors, liquids, and dissolved ionic and nonionic solutes is presented. The historical preface is followed by a discussion of the limiting transport mechanism in consolidated and microporous membranes, respectively.

The important phenomena of ultrafiltration and reverse osmosis (hyperfiltration) are treated in detail. Specific technological limitations of these processes are acknowledged and explained. Donnan's exclusion effects in ion-selective membranes are discussed briefly.

Various medical and pharmaceutical applications of membrane science including blood oxygenation, hemodialysis, blood ultrafiltration, serum concentration, controlled and sustained drug release to various organs, and barrier materials for pharmaceutical packaging are discussed in light of the limiting transport mechanisms and the various membrane processes.

REFERENCES

1.   Choo, C. Y., Bixler, H. J., Michaels, A. S., and Baddour, R. F., Ind. Eng. Chem. Proc. Des. Dev., 1, 14 (1962).

2.   Michaels, A. S., Chem. Eng. Prog., 64, 31 (1968).

3.   Loeb, S. and Sourirajan, S., U. S. Patent 3,133,132 (1964).

4.   Mahon, H. I., Proceedings of the Desalination Research Conference, Publication No. 942, National Academy of Sciences, Washington, D.C., 1963, p. 345.

5.   Stannett, V. T., in Diffusion in Polymers, J. Crank and
     G. S. Park, Eds., Academic Press, London and New York,
     1967, p. 41.

6.   Merten, U., Ed., Desalination by Reverse Osmosis, MIT
     Press, Cambridge, Mass., 1966.

7.   Thomas, D. G., Griffith, W. L., and Keller, R. M.,
     Desalination, 9, 33 (1971).

8.   Blatt, W. F., Dravid, A., Michaels, A. S. and Nelson, L.,
     in Membrane Science and Technology: Industrial, Biological,
     and Waste Treatment Processes, J. E. Flinn, Ed., Plenum
     Press, New York, 1970, p. 47.

9.   Michaels, A. S., Chem. Eng. Prog., 64, 31 (1968).

10. Michaels, A. S., Bixler, H. J., and Hodges, R. M., Jr.,
     J. Colloid Sci., 20, 1034 (1965).

11. Kesting, R. E., Subcasky, W. J. and Paton, J. D., J.
     Colloid Interface Sci., 28, 156 (1968).

12. Palmer, J. A., Hopfenberg, H. B., and Felder, R. M.,
     ibid., 45, 223 (1973).

13. Bailey, M. W., Hopfenberg, H. B., and Stannett, V.,
     presented at the 74th National Meeting of the American
     Institute of Chemical Engineers, New Orleans, La.,
     March 11-15, 1973.

14. Donnan, F. G., Elektrochem. Z., 17, 572 (1911).

15. Lonsdale, H. K., Pusch, W., and Walch, A., Trans.
     Faraday Soc. (in press).

16. Blatt, W. F., Feinberg, M. P., Hopfenberg, H. B., and
     Saravis, C. A., Science, 150, 224 (1965).

17. Porter, M. C. and Nelson, L., in Recent Developments
     in Separation Science: Interfacial Phenomena in Fluid
     Phase Separation Processes, Vol. II, N. N. Li, Ed., CRC
     Press, Cleveland, Ohio, 1972, p. 227.

COLLAGEN: A BIOLOGICAL PLASTIC

Kurt H. Stenzel, Teruo Miyata, and
Albert L. Rubin

Rogosin Kidney Center, The New York Hospital-
Cornell Medical Center, New York, New York

Collagen is, in many ways, a biological plastic. The dictionary definition of plastic includes such phrases as, it "suggests qualities, such as those of wax or clay, soft enough to be molded yet capable of hardening into desired form". Collagen is synthesized in certain specialized animal cells as a soluble material which is then secreted from the cell and hardened by a variety of poorly understood control mechanisms. This results in collagen materials for the function, support, and protection of various animal organs. Our interest has been, first, to understand the structure of this material and its importance in medicine and biology; and, second, to isolate, purify, and restructure collagen as a possible replacement for damaged organs or tissues. A protein that comprises more than 25% of human tissues is, of course, of great interest to medical scientists. Alterations of collagenous materials in disease are of profound importance in understanding many pathological processes. Since there is always room for improvement of artificial organs, investigation of the properties of a natural biomaterial is also of value.

STRUCTURE AND SYNTHESIS OF COLLAGEN

Collagen molecules are organized in a very precise way in most fibrous tissues: each molecule is aligned end-to-end with another, and the molecules are polymerized side-to-side in a quarter-stagger arrangement [1]. Acid-soluble collagen has been used in most studies dealing with the structure of collagen molecules. Small amounts of collagen can be isolated from skin or tendon by extraction with dilute acid, and the solubilized collagen can be purified by reprecipitation. Acid-soluble collagen accounts for only 3-5% of the total collagen of connective tissue. The isolated collagen molecule, tropocollagen, consists of three polypeptide chains. The entire molecule has a molecular weight of about 300,000 and each subunit peptide has a molecular weight of about 100,000 [2]. The chains are organized as a triple helix and are stabilized primarily by hydrogen bonds. Upon denaturation, a further differentiation of collagen can be detected. When collagen is denatured, the triple-helical structure is lost, and the individual polypeptide chains assume a random-coil configuration. Denaturation occurs at low temperatures (about 40°C) and this characteristic of collagen has been used for centuries to extract gelatin from animal connective tissue [3]. Covalent bonds occur between polypeptide chains in some types of collagen; these can link either two or all three chains together. Collagen with no intermolecular crosslinks is known as "alpha-collagen"; with two polypeptide chains linked together, as "beta-collagen"; and when all three chains are crosslinked, the material is known as "gamma-collagen". There is generally a higher concentration of gamma-collagen in preparations from older individuals.

Because of the marked asymmetry of collagen molecules, 2800 Å long and 15 Å wide, they have a high viscosity in relatively dilute solutions, and they also tend to aggregate spontaneously and form fibers under physiologic conditions. Some years ago, Professor Schmitt's group at MIT investigated the effect of proteolytic enzymes on tropocollagen [4]. They found that treatment with pepsin does not destroy the triple helix, but that it does alter the interaction properties of collagen. When tropocollagen in acid solution is dialyzed against water, the molecules spontaneously undergo linear polymerization and the viscosity of the solution increases sharply. If the collagen is first treated with pepsin, however, this linear polymerization occurs to a considerably lesser degree. Pepsin treatment also affects the intermolecular bonding in that there tends to be a change from beta- to alpha-collagen, as seen both on column chromatography and ultracentrifugation. These studies, of course, depend upon complete removal of the enzyme prior to subjecting collagen to denaturing conditions. When collagen is denatured, it becomes susceptible to proteolytic enzymes. The enzyme can be removed from the collagen by free diffusion electrophoresis. Separation of the peptides resulting from pepsin treatment of collagen shows that they have a different overall makeup from those of the bulk of the triple-helical tropocollagen. The conclusions reached from these studies are that collagen contains nonhelical peptides which are susceptible to proteolytic digestion and that these nonhelical appendages are important determinants of both intra- and intermolecular crosslinks [5].

Dr. Nishihara and others [6] found that most insoluble collagen could be solubilized with proteolytic enzymes. The solubilized material could easily be purified and was found to retain many of the molecular properties of native collagen. This is the material that we have used for most of our studies on biomaterials.

There are two major types of subunit polypeptide chains of collagen, termed the "alpha-1" and "alpha-2" chain [7]. Most collagen from skin and tendon consists of two alpha-1 and one alpha-2 chains. Cyanogen bromide treatment cleaves the collagen chains into 5-9 subunits, and these peptides have been used for the study of the primary structure of collagen [8]. The amino acid composition of collagen includes a high percentage of glycine (about 33%) and of hydroxyproline and hydroxylysine. There are many imino acids and these probably account for the triple-helical structure of collagen. The typical repeating sequence in collagen is $(Gly-X-Y)_n$.

The intramolecular crosslinks found in nature, which are so difficult to rupture other than by proteolytic attack, are due to the enzymatic oxidation of lysine and hydroxylysine residues to collagen aldehydes. These then react with other aldehydes or free amino groups on neighboring molecules [9].

Collagen is synthesized on polysomes of the endoplasmic reticulum, mainly in fibroblasts, but probably in other cells as well. Proline and lysine are enzymatically hydroxylated after the polypeptide chains have been released in the intracellular matrix. Carbohydrate is then added to the hydroxylysine residues, and the molecule assumes a triple-helical configuration. It is soluble at this stage, has a higher molecular weight than tropocollagen, and is secreted from the cell in this form. Specific peptidases digest portions of the nonhelical segments of this procollagen in extracellular sites, and this leads to mature tropocollagen. Enzymatic polymerization of the molecule then occurs [10]. Degradation of collagen is largely the result of a specific enzyme "collagenase".

This is the only proteolytic enzyme known that can digest the triple-helical portion of collagen [11].

MEDICAL AND BIOLOGICAL SIGNIFICANCE

Collagen has been used as a biomaterial in both its native form and as resolubilized and restructured materials. The most successful native materials used in clinical medicine are bovine carotid heterografts [12]. These are prepared commercially by Johnson & Johnson by treating carefully cleaned bovine carotid arteries with a proteolytic enzyme, ficin, and crosslinking them with an aldehyde, dialdehyde starch. These materials are certainly not pure collagen; they contain other connective tissue elements as well. In our clinical service, these grafts are used extensively for blood access in patients on hemodialysis. Many patients, especially diabetics, have poor blood vessels, and it is difficult to create either fistulas or shunts. For these individuals, bovine grafts work well; the grafts are large, they can be punctured almost immediately and for innumerable times thereafter, and there is a very low incidence of occlusion by thrombus formation.

We have been interested in restructuring purified enzyme-solubilized collagen and evaluating these kinds of materials. One of the simplest experiments is to prepare films of collagen, crosslink them in a variety of ways, and determine their physical and biological properties. The results of these studies indicate that collagen films, crosslinked with glutaraldehyde, have an increased denaturation temperature (from 40°C in control films up to 90°C with crosslinked films) and that they are remarkably resistant to bacterial collagenase. Films have been implanted in a variety of sites in rabbits, and they last for prolonged periods of time with minimal inflammatory reaction [13].

Effects of collagen films on blood are of great importance. Collagen is a potent material for initiation of platelet aggregation [14], and recent studies by Jaffe, et al. [15] indicate that the collagen must be organized with a particular macromolecular architecture for this agglutination to take place. The interactions of collagen and platelets are important in both the medical and biomaterials aspects of collagen. Many kinds of tissue injury could be initiated by endothelial damage and subsequent interaction between the underlying basement membrane (of which collagen is a prominent component) and the blood.

Enzyme-solubilized and restructured collagen appears to have a minimal affinity for platelets. We dialyzed both dogs and humans against collagen membranes, and scanning electron micrographs of the surfaces were done by A. Schwartz at Cornell University [16]. We found that, in normal dogs, platelets adhere almost selectively to cuprophane membranes; collagen, however, binds only small numbers of a variety of cell types, including some platelets and some white cells. When anemic humans are dialyzed, the cuprophane membranes tend to accumulate large numbers of white cells rather than platelets (predominately polymorphonuclear leucocytes), whereas collagen membranes again have a variety of cell types on their surfaces but not to the degree that cuprophane does. Some attempts were also made to elute proteins from both cuprophane and collagen membranes after perfusion with blood. The initial results indicate that more serum protein is adsorbed onto the collagen than onto cuprophane surfaces. The adsorbed material appears to be one component which migrates like albumin on disc electrophoresis.

Antigenicity is another problem that must be dealt with in using natural biomaterials. Collagen is a difficult antigen to study because of its poor solubility, but several investigators have been able to identify antigenic sites on collagen by passive hemagglutination and complement fixation techniques [17]. Moreover, the use of such materials as bovine heterografts has apparently not resulted in adverse immunologic effects [18]. We have been unable to detect antibodies in our studies after implanting collagen into animals. Antibodies can be found if the collagen is injected repeatedly along with Freund's adjuvant. The final importance of this factor, however, in the use of collagen materials remains to be determined.

Collagen has been tried as a material for many uses in medicine, including a hemostatic agent where native collagen is prepared as a very fine powder [19], a covering for burn dressings [20], a replacement for dura mater [21], hemodialysis membranes [22], a replacement for blood vessels [23], and heart valves [24], and various treatment devices for eye diseases. Some of the eye applications illustrate general aspects of the use of collagen as a biomaterial.

Collagen can be used to replace the vitreous body of the eye. The vitreous is often damaged, especially in diabetes and other diseases, by hemorrhage. In these situations, the vitreous can sometimes be removed and replaced with another material. Collagen has been used for this [25], but occasionally even enzyme-solubilized and irradiated collagen becomes opaque after some time [26]. An important aspect of the plasticity of collagen is the fact that collagen can be altered by a variety of techniques and its physical properties changed to meet specific medical requirements. When collagen is placed in the vitreous, it should not form fibers since this leads to opacification. Succinylation of free amino groups of collagen results in a protein having many free carboxyl groups [27]. This material is soluble at physiologic pH, and so should not form fibers in the vitreous body. Succinylated collagen can be crosslinked by gamma-irradiation to give it the desired viscosity.

Collagen membranes inserted in the lamellae of the cornea last for many years and are gradually resorbed and replaced by what is apparently normal corneal tissue [28]. This is unusual for materials placed in the cornea: most are extruded as foreign bodies.

Collagen may also be used as a vehicle for drug delivery [29]. We have employed collagen-pilocarpine films in the treatment of glaucoma [30]. Collagen and pilocarpine are mixed; films are prepared and then cut to appropriate size. In vitro studies show that release of the drug is retarded, and in vivo studies in rabbits indicate prolonged physiological activity. Initial studies in patients with glaucoma [31] have resulted in 24-hour control of intraocular pressure in most patients. The drug is simply entrapped in the collagen film for this application, and the drug release, which is probably completed within half an hour, suffices to control intraocular pressure. The collagen then dissolves, and the patient is not encumbered by any further foreign body in the eye.

Many drugs are water-soluble and diffuse rapidly out of collagen matrices. A method for crosslinking collagen-drug combinations has been developed in experiments designed to immobilize heparin in collagen materials. Since collagen binds heparin at low pH, collagen-heparin films were prepared at pH 3.4. To prevent removal of heparin during crosslinking, glutaraldehyde was diluted with ethanol. Heparin is insoluble in this solution, and the desired degree of crosslinking can be obtained. These films markedly prolong the release of heparin, from several minutes for control films to several weeks for crosslinked ones [32].

Biologic modifications of collagen, i.e., those occurring in nature, are extensive. They indicate the wide variety of materials that can be made from collagen. The enclosure and regulation of an internal environment was one of the most important steps in the evolution of vertebrates [33]. It allowed them to be free of the primordial seas, and it allowed successive orders of vertebrates to attain biologic prominence. The kidneys regulate this internal environment, but collagen encloses it and protects it from the vicissitudes of the external environment. We can live in a desert or a jungle, or swim in salt or fresh water, and our body fluids remain protected. Such diverse structures as bone, skin, tendons, and basement membranes contain collagen as the major structural protein.

Basement membrane is one of the most interesting and one of the least understood of the connective tissues. The collagen component is not fibrous, and the typical 690 Å collagen band pattern cannot be identified [34]. Recent studies have shown that this collagen is highly insoluble, might be linked to other basement membrane components by disulfide bridges, contains more carbohydrates than other collagens, and consists solely of alpha-1 chains. Further knowledge of this ubiquitous membrane should lead to a greater understanding of disease and could lead to new biomaterials applications.

SUMMARY

The study of collagen, despite our broad knowledge of the molecular structure of this protein, is still in its infancy. This is especially true in terms of the medical aspects of collagen. A greater understanding of modified collagen and of ways of cross-linking the material will be of great value in using collagen in various surgical procedures. Certainly the collagens are not in competition with synthetic materials; they are simply different and may have different applications. To those primarily interested in medicine, collagen has a tremendous appeal because of its widespread occurrence and its importance in many pathological processes.

ACKNOWLEDGMENTS

Supported in part by grants from the National Science Foundation and the John A. Hartford Foundation.

REFERENCES

1.   Hodge, A. J. and Schmitt, F. O., Proc. Nat. Acad. Sci. USA, 46, 186 (1960).

2.   Gallop, P. M., Blumenfeld, O. O., and Seifter, S., Ann. Rev. Biochem., 41, 617 (1972).

3.   Piez, K. A., ibid., 37, 547 (1968).

4.   Hodge, A. J., Highberger, J. H., Defner, G.G.J., and Schmitt, F. O., Proc. Nat. Acad. Sci. USA, 46, 197 (1960).

5.   Rubin, A. L., Pfahl, D., Speakman, P. T., Davison, P. F., and Schmitt, F. O., Science, 13, 37 (1963).

6.   Nishihara, T. and Miyata T., Collagen Symp. (Japan), 3, 66 (1962).

7.   Piez, K. A., in Treatise on Collagen, G. N. Ramachandran, Ed., Vol. I, Academic Press, London and New York, 1967, pp. 207-252.

8.   Traub, W. and Piez, K. A., Advan. Protein Chem., 25, 243 (1971).

9.   Tanzer, M. L., Science, 180, 561 (1973).

10. Grant, M. E. and Prockop, D. J., New Engl. J. Med., 286, 194-99, 242-49, 291-300 (1972).

11. Mandl, I., Ed., Collagenase: 1st Interdisciplinary Symposium, Columbia University, College of Physicians and Surgeons, 1970, Gordon and Breach, New York, 1972.

12. Rosenberg, N., Lord, G. H., Henderson, J., Bothwell, J. W., and Gaughran, E.R.L., Surgery, 65, 951 (1970).

13.   White, M. J., Kohno, I., Rubin, A. L., Stenzel, K. H., and Miyata, T., Biomater., Med. Devices, Artif. Organs, 1, 703 (1973).

14.   Wilner, G. D., Nossel, H. L., and LeRoy, E. C., J. Clin. Invest., 47, 2616 (1968).

15.   Jaffe, R., and Deykin, D., ibid., 53, 875 (1974).

16.   Schwartz, A., Ast, D., Kohno, I., Stenzel, K. H., and Rubin, A. L., Abstracts, Annual Meeting of American Society of Biological Chemists and Biophysical Society, Minneapolis, Minn., June 2-7, 1974.

17.   Timpl, R., Wolff, I., Wick, G., Furthmayr, H., and Steffen, C., J. Immunol., 101, 725 (1968).

18.   DeFalco, R. J., J. Surg. Res., 10, 95 (1970).

19.   Hait, M. P., Amer. J. Surg., 120, 330 (1970).

20.   Sakurai, I. and Miyata, T., personal communication.

21.   Kline, D. G., Arch. Surg., 91, 924 (1965).

22.   Stenzel, K. H., Rubin, A. L., Yamayoshi, W., Miyata, T., Suzuki, T., Sohde, T., and Nishizawa, M., Trans. Amer. Soc. Artif. Intern. Organs, 17, 293 (1971).

23.   Chvapil, M. and Krajicek, M., Mod. Trends Vasc. Surg., 1, 120 (1970).

24.   Carpentier, A., et al., J. Thorac. Cardiov. Surg., 62, 707 (1971).

25.   Dunn, M. W., Shaffer, D., Stenzel, K. H., Miyata, T., Hopkins, L. E., and Powers, M. J., Trans. Amer. Soc. Artif. Intern. Organs, 17, 421 (1971).

26.   Pruett, R. C., Calabria, G. A., and Schepens, C. L., Arch. Ophthalmol., 88, 840 (1972).

27.   Olcott, H. S. and Fraenkel-Conrat, H., Chem. Rev., 41, 151 (1947).

28.   Dunn, M. W., Stenzel, K. H., Hopkins, L. E., Powers,
      M. J., Rubin, A. L., and Miyata, T., J. Ophthal. Surg.,
      2, 1 (1971).

29.   Horakova, Z., Krajicek, M., Chvapil, M., and Boissier, J.,
      Therapie, 22, 1455 (1967).

30.   Rubin, A. L., Stenzel, K. H., Miyata, T., White, M. J.,
      and Dunn, M., J. Clin. Pharmacol., 13, 309 (1973).

31.   Dunn, M. W., personal communication.

32.   Miyata, T., personal communication.

33.   Smith, H., From Fish to Philosopher, Doubleday, Anchor,
      Garden City, N. Y., 1961.

34.   Kefalides, N. A., Int. Rev. Connect. Tissue Res. 6, 63
      (1973).

BIODEGRADABLE POLYMERS IN MEDICINE AND SURGERY

Richard L. Kronenthal

Ethicon, Inc., Somerville, New Jersey 08876

INTRODUCTION

The science of biodegradable materials is most often associated with problems of environmental control. The need to avoid accumulation of permanent ecological litter is obvious and methods to do so will not be considered in this discussion. Rather, the emphasis will be on polymers with the potential for degradation within the living organism. More specifically, polymers which display structural integrity and, as a consequence, mechanical utility, will be considered while polymeric drugs or carriers which function in solution, such as polyvinyl pyrollidone and dextran, both reported as useful blood extenders, will not.

THE PHENOMENA OF DEGRADATION

Before describing the various classes of materials that have been utilized in medicine and surgery, some discussion of the general manner by which most polymers degrade in the tissue environment would be useful. With few exceptions, the common belief that polymers simply erode away like a slowly dissolving crystal while maintaining their initial strength and integrity in the residual mass is not correct. When first inserted in the aqueous environment of the body, polymers may be considered to undergo four stages of degradation (Table I). The first, hydration, is variable in rate, degree and effect, and is dependent upon the

119

TABLE I

FOUR STAGES OF POLYMER DEGRADATION
IN VIVO

---

1. Hydration -   Disruption of van der Waals'
                                   forces and hydrogen bonds.

2. Strength Loss -   Initial cleavage of backbone
                                   covalent bonds.

3. Loss of Mass Integrity -   Further cleavage of covalent
                                   bonds to polymer molecular
                                   weight levels insufficient for
                                   mass coherence.

4. Mass Loss -   Dissolution of low molecular
   (Solubilization)   weight species and phagocyto-
                                   sis of small fragments.

nature of the polymer. Natural polymers such as collagen rapidly absorb appreciable quantities of water so that there is an almost immediate and significant reduction in strength compared to the unimplanted control. Other materials, such as polyglycolide, absorb little water and display negligible changes in physical properties during the hydration stage. This stage of absorption may be considered complete within minutes or hours after implantation unless, of course, the implant volume is so large that the diffusion of water into the mass simply takes longer. During this stage, few, if any, covalent bonds are broken. The primary effects result from disruption of secondary and tertiary structures stabilized by van der Waal's forces and hydrogen bonds.

The second stage of degradation is manifested by the irreversible loss of implant strength, usually as a result of covalent bond cleavage involving the polymer backbone. This is a most interesting stage which can be mediated by a number of mechanisms, depending upon the polymer. For example, using histochemical methods, Salthouse, et al. [1] have shown that, for collagen, several enzyme systems sequentially attack the protein. Other work[2] revealed that the rate of lysosomal enzyme attack on the reconstituted collagen molecule backbone is affected by, and can be regulated by the disposition of the side chain amino groups of certain basic amino acids. In fact, if most such groups are blocked, even without crosslinking, undenatured collagen can be transformed into an essentially nonabsorbable protein retaining most of its original strength over long periods of in vivo residence [3]. Apparently, amino groups are required for enzymic coordination prior to peptide bond cleavage, and their alteration with blocking agents prevents or significantly retards normal enzymic degradation.

In the case of absorbable polyesters, the rate of strength loss is governed entirely by the rate of simple hydrolytic cleavage of the polymer backbone and is independent of any known enzyme systems. In this class of polymers, the strength loss rate is dependent upon temperature, pH, and especially upon the degree of crystallinity of the polymer. More highly crystalline species may be expected to maintain their strength for longer periods of time compared to those which are more amorphous, and the classical situation of hydrolytic tie molecule breakage in amorphous regions between crystallites would appear to be operative in the degradation of this type of material.

The third stage of degradation involves the beginning of the absorptive or mass loss process. In what may be considered to be continuation of Stage 2 covalent bond breaking, the polymer is degraded to a molecular weight level below that required for coherence, and a friable or gelatinized mass which may fragment or partially solubilize results. The actual molecular weight reduction necessary to reach this stage depends upon many factors, polymer conformation and crystallinity to mention two, and is not easily defined in specific terms. It should be emphasized, however, that at the end of Stage 2, most or all of the original mass is still present and that it is only during and after Stage 3 that actual mass loss or absorption occurs.

The complete removal of polymer from the tissue may be considered as the fourth stage of absorption. The polymer may lose mass simply by the solubilization of low molecular weight species into the intercellular fluid. Alternatively, small fragments may be removed from the implant site by phagocytes and eventually carried to the lymphatic system for completion of the solubilization process. This stage of absorption may occur without apparent histological change for an extended period, if the original form of the polymer is without physical disruption and if solubilization occurs uniformly throughout the mass. In this situation, the density of the mass decreases as solubilization proceeds until a "ghost" of the original implant is all that remains. Eventually the ghost is also absorbed.

It is obvious that the absorption processes just described apply to truly biodegradable polymers in the sense that they are depolymerized and the products of depolymerization as such or as metabolized fragments are eliminated from the body. It is also possible that polymeric masses may be removed from implant sites without actual reduction in the chain length through solubilization processes involving side chain modification rather than backbone scission. For example, the reported absorption of polyvinyl alcohol derivatives may be considered to occur through the hydrolysis of acetate side groups to produce the more hydrophilic and, therefore, more soluble alcohol. In this case, it is doubtful that mechanisms exist for the metabolic cleavage of the substituted polymethylene polymer chains. A possible exception to the reported stability of polymethylene derivatives involves the alkyl cyanoacrylate tissue adhesives which form highly polarized polymers exhibiting reduced electron density on alternate backbone carbon atoms and which have been postulated to undergo a reverse Knoevenagel condensation reaction resulting in polymethylene backbone scission [4]. It is difficult to visualize how polymethylene polymers can be eliminated from the body without a mechanism of this type although it is possible that solubilized but molecularly undegraded materials of such nature reside invisibly, benignly, and permanently in the tissues.

BIODEGRADABLE SYNTHETIC POLYMERS

No attempt will be made to include all the systems reported to be biodegradable. Rather, the major classes of polymers will be considered together with some selected unique systems.

In the preceding presentation and elsewhere [3], applications of collagen in medicine and surgery have been described. The use of collagen in reconstructive and other surgery has been seriously explored in many laboratories because collagen combines many of the factors necessary for a suitable biodegradable implant. Table II lists six primary characteristics required for a successful implant. It is the combination of these properties in one substance

TABLE II

CHARACTERISTICS OF A SUCCESSFUL
BIODEGRADABLE IMPLANT

---

1. Formability
2. Adequate initial strength and dimensional stability
3. Controlled rate of strength loss
4. Complete absorbability
5. Low order of toxicity of both implant
   and degradation products
6. Sterilizability

that provides the unique properties of a useful biodegradable
system. Toxicity, as used here, includes frank tissue irritation
as well as the more subacute characteristics, such as carcino-
genicity, immunogenicity, teratologic effects, etc. Collagen, the
major connective tissue protein, has found wide application as a
surgical suture in the form of catgut as well as purified reconstituted fibers, and well fulfills the six basic requirements listed in
Table II. Its properties have served as a model for the development of other biodegradable materials and, on this basis, it is not
difficult to understand why some of the earliest work in synthetic
biodegradable polymer development involved polymers containing
the peptide linkage.

Polyamino Acids

Many different polyamino acids have been synthesized, primarily as models for studying proteins, and some of these polymers have been shown to be fibrous.

Studies on polyglutamates and polyglutamic acid revealed that
these substances were not sufficiently strong to be considered for
use as absorbable surgical sutures [5]. Generally, polyglutamic
acid is a relatively weak material which loses strength and solu-
bilizes within a few days after implantation. On the other hand,
the corresponding methyl and benzyl esters have appreciable
long-term strength in vivo, but are not sufficiently absorbable.

Miyamae and his co-workers [6] found that partial esterification with lower alcohols of the polyglutamic acid residues in fibers prepared by extruding the sodium salt of this polyamino acid provided the requisite combination of strength and absorbability. However, as with most of the polypeptides, the maximum achievable strength was significantly lower than that of collagen and some of the synthetic absorbable fibers. This does not, of course preclude other applications of these materials, for example, as drug release vehicles where high strength is not mandatory.

Randall [7], working in England, found that copolymerization of an L-imino acid such as proline with an L-amino acid such as glutamic acid resulted in fibrous synthetic polypeptides. These polymers were prepared by the random copolymerization of the respective N-carboxyanhydride derivatives of the amino acids and were claimed to be useful as absorbable sutures. Poly-β-alanine is not an α-polyamino acid, but was found to form filaments by either wet or dry spinning when combined with formic acid [8].

Goodman, et al. [9] reported that linear polydepsipeptide copolymers derived from α-, β-, and γ-hydroxy as well as α-amino acids, were fiber- and film-forming materials which were easily hydrolyzed and thus were applicable as synthetic absorbable substances. Figure 1 illustrates the synthetic routes involved. Copolymers of α-amino acids with α-hydroxyacids are prepared by copolymerizing the corresponding N-carboxyanhydrides and anhydrosulfites, while the inclusion of β-hydroxy acids is achieved through the copolymerization of the N-carboxyanhydride with the corresponding lactone.

Polyvinyl Alcohol Derivatives

Polyvinyl alcohol has been the base for several materials claimed to be absorbable. However, as stated previously, the definitive research required to demonstrate the metabolic fate of this family of polymers has yet to be done.

Reports on the use of polyvinyl alcohol derivatives for surgical devices and sutures are numerous although few details concerning the biological responses to these materials have been described. Nachinkin, et al. [10] reported that polyvinyl alcohol fibers which

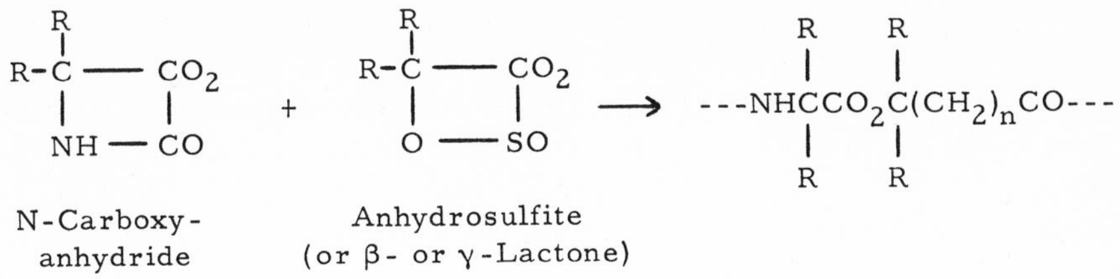

$$\begin{array}{ccc}
\overset{R}{\underset{NH-CO}{\overset{|}{R-C}}\!\!-\!\!CO_2} & + & \overset{R}{\underset{O-SO}{\overset{|}{R-C}}\!\!-\!\!CO_2} & \longrightarrow & ---NHCCO_2C(CH_2)_nCO---
\end{array}$$

FIGURE 1. Polydepsipeptide synthesis.

were crosslinked with formaldehyde possessed increased dimensional stability. These workers describe the "absorption" of this material in terms of fragmentation into small particles and it is questionable if Stage 4 absorption ever occurred.

Shelton and Thompson [11] pointed out the need for heating completely deacetylated polyvinyl alcohol to impart strength and dimensional stability to the product. Other workers [12, 13] combined polyvinyl alcohol with various polymers such as cellulose, starch, gelatin and albumin, as well as with small molecule organic acids, and reported improved absorbability. These findings may be explained by visualizing a more rapid physical disintegration of the implant rather than actual mass disappearance.

Mirkovitch and his co-workers [14] reported on the biological fate of plate-cast polyvinyl alcohol sutures used in bronchial, gastrointestinal and vascular surgery. Little tissue reaction was produced compared to catgut. The tensile strength decreased to about one-third of its original value after four months and about 20% of the original strength was retained after one year. The sutures were still present macroscopically at that time so that, again, the true absorbability of these materials could be questioned.

Sutures based on polyvinyl alcohol have been marketed commercially in Japan as synthetic catgut.

Fritsch [15] reported that polyvinyl butyral was rapidly degradable and comparable to catgut in this respect. Its use as an absorbable suture was proposed. Except for the Japanese product, no suture based on reportedly absorbable polyvinyl alcohol polymers has ever been marketed.

β-Polyesters

Two polymers especially prepared as absorbable materials are poly-β-propiolactone [16] and poly-β-hydroxybutyrate [17]. Propiolactone was polymerized by subjecting the monomer to ionizing radiation whereas the butyrate polymer was obtained from cultures of a microorganism. Intramuscular implants of β-hydroxybutyrate were reported to begin to dissolve after eight weeks. The propiolactone derivative did indeed lose strength in vivo, but Stage 4 absorption was found not to occur within a period of several months [18].

α-Polyester Homopolymers

The simplest α-polyester is polyglycolide or polyglycolic acid. It is conveniently synthesized from a glycolide melt through a salt-catalyzed ring-opening mechanism according to Figure 2.

Numerous other methods for the synthesis of polyglycolic acid and closely related systems have also been reported. Frazza and

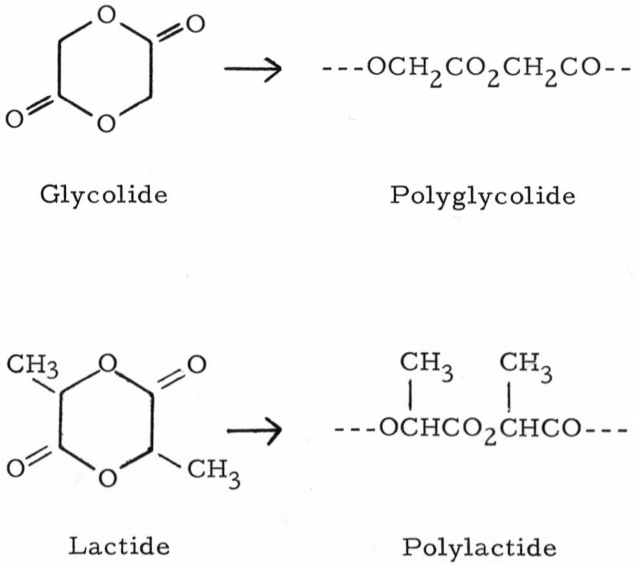

Glycolide   Polyglycolide

Lactide   Polylactide

FIGURE 2. Synthesis of polyglycolide and polylactide.

Schmitt [19] have described the development of commercial methods for preparing polyglycolide fibers of value as synthetic absorbable sutures and many clinical papers have appeared on the surgical utilization of this material as sutures and ligatures in a variety of tissues.

Braided sutures prepared from polyglycolide were reported to exhibit high strength, excellent handling properties, minimal tissue reactivity and an absorption profile similar to that of catgut.

Reports on the utilization of polyglycolide in prosthetic devices include the fabrication of a tracheal replacement based on dip-coating a porous wire mesh with polymer [20]. Fabrication of films, fabrics and solid forms from polyglycolide has also been described [21].

An unusual application of polyglycolide was suggested by Semp [22]. The finely powdered polymer was found to be an effective lubricant for surgical gloves, tubing, and drains. In the event of accidental transfer of the powder to internal sites, the effect of adverse tissue reaction was claimed to be minimized compared to conventional starch-based lubricants. Schmitt, et al. [23] applied the same principle used by Kim, et al. [24] for creating biodegradable polymers through the inclusion of hydrolyzable blocks. In this case, blocks of polyglycolide representing 5-15% of the total polymer weight are incorporated into a variety of otherwise stable polymers. For example, the lability of poly-ϵ-caprolactone to attack by water was significantly increased by blocking with polyglycolide or polylactide.

Polylactide or polylactic acid may be considered as an oxygen analogue of polyalanine just as polyglycolide is related to polyglycine, and is prepared by polymerizing lactide (Fig. 2). The kinetics and mechanisms of this synthesis have been studied by Dittrich, et al. [25].

Methods for the synthesis of polylactide have been reported by many workers including Higgins [26] and even block copolymers with epichlorohydrin have been prepared [27] in an effort to produce a material with less hydrolytic lability than polylactide. Flory, et al. [28, 29] have studied the configuration of random polylactide chains and Mhala and Mishra [30] have investigated the kinetics of hydrolysis of D, L-lactide as well as lactyl lactic acid.

Kulkarni and his co-workers [31, 32] were among the first to describe the use of polylactide for surgical implants. Polylactide was prepared from both L(+)- and D, L-lactic acid and converted into films, coatings and fibers. Low inflammatory responses were observed throughout the six-week observation period, after which time most of the polymer remained. In vivo studies utilizing ^{14}C-labeled polymer showed a 14% loss of mass after three months, indicating a relatively slow rate of absorption compared to polyglycolide. No residual systemic radioactivity was found, showing complete metabolic conversion to carbon dioxide. These workers also compared the kinetics of degradation of the D, L- and L(-)- polymers and found that the D, L form degraded more rapidly. This is not unexpected because the optically active polymer displays a higher order of crystallinity and suggests that copolymers of D, L- and L(-)-lactide can be utilized to control degradation rate.

One problem existing with the D, L polymer is its dimensional instability as manifested by shrinkage after implantation in tissue. Hodge [33] attempted to stabilize a monofilament made of this polymer by subjecting it to heat, stretching and radiation. None of these treatments was successful.

Fouty [34] and Schneider [35] have both described the preparation of high molecular weight polylactides for use as surgical sutures, and Schneider [36] has proposed the use of fabric grafts of polylactide for surgical reconstruction. Such materials were evaluated as tracheal prostheses by Thomas [37], who found that polylactide demonstrated increased tissue response and fibroplasia compared to nonabsorbable polyester (Dacron) prostheses which were said to be more acceptable.

Getter, et al. [38] evaluated polylactic acid in the form of plates and screws for the repair of canine mandibular fractures. The implants were found to be partially degraded after six weeks and completely absorbed after 32 weeks. The fracture sites, at that time, were indistinguishable from adjacent bony areas.

Cutright, et al. [39] employed sheets of polylactic acid to repair blowout fractures of the orbital floor in monkeys. The animals were followed for 38 weeks, at which time it was found that the implants were well tolerated but not completely absorbed although phagocytosis of polymer fragments was occurring. Cutright and co-workers [40] also studied the degradation of

polylactic acid sutures in rats and found gradual degradation lasting beyond the 90-day observation period. Gregory, et al. [41]
prepared and evaluated polylactic acid films as burn dressings; at
thicknesses required to control water loss, polylactic acid was
found to be too stiff and unconforming to be of value in this application.

Several studies have been completed on the absorption mechanism of polylactide. Brady, et al [42] implanted ^{14}C-labeled
polylactide in rats and assayed urine, feces and respired air for
radioactivity for 168 days, after which time 63% of the original
implant remained. Degradation was linear and about 29% of the
radioactivity was eliminated as carbon dioxide via the respiratory
system rather than through the urine or feces. This finding compared favorably with that of Hegyeli [43], who measured the rate
of degradation of polylactic acid in vitro using chick embryo organ
homogenates maintained in tissue culture media. This method was
proposed as being generally applicable to the assay of biodegradability of polymer systems.

Polylactides have been proposed as carriers for drugs.
Jackanicz, et al. [44] have measured the rate of release of
norgestrel from poly-L-lactic acid films in vivo and in vitro.
Films, 2.5 mils thick, containing 33% norgestrel released about
3 mg/day/sq cm over an 80-day period. Subcutaneous implants
in rats initially released 5.5 mg/day/sq cm of drug which declined
to 3 mg/day/sq cm by 80 days. During this time, the polylactide
matrix lost coherence and began to shrink and fragment. A very
low order of tissue reactivity was elicited. These workers point
out the desirability of having the carrier degrade at the same rate
that the drug is released so that the carrier and the drug will
"disappear" together. It is not likely that this can be easily
achieved because of the variability of the systems involved, and
it would appear that as long as the carrier does not invoke adverse
reactions, its presence in tissue for a reasonable period after the
drug has been exhausted would not be of significance.

Boswell, et al. [45] have described poly-L-lactide, poly-
D, L-lactide as well as copolymers of lactide and glycolide as
carriers for drugs, particularly 17-β-estradiol at levels between
5% and 25%. The mixture was compressed into tablets suitable
for parenteral administration. The application of this system for
hormone replacement therapy was cited.

α-Polyester Copolymers

Polyglycolides are highly crystalline materials which undergo relatively rapid in vivo degradation. Polylactides, on the other hand, remain in tissue for extended periods depending, in part, on whether the optically active or racemic monomer is used. However, as mentioned previously, poly-D,L-lactide displays comparatively lower tensile strength and poorer dimensional stability. Wasserman and Levy [46] have approached this problem by preparing copolymers of glycolide and lactide as shown in Figure 3. It has been found that fibers suitable as synthetic absorbable sutures can be prepared utilizing a 10:90 weight percent ratio of lactide and glycolide. This copolymer displays less crystallinity than homopolyglycolide and is said to retain its tensile strength longer and absorb more rapidly than homopolyglycolide.

Cutright, et al. [47] compared pellets of polylactide, polyglycolide, and copolymers of 75:25, 50:50, and 25:75 lactide and glycolide. The pellets were implanted in rat femurs and harvested over a 220-day period. The 25% lactide copolymer degraded first followed, in order, by 50%, 75% and then polylactide which degraded most slowly of all the samples studied. It should be noted that these measurements were histological estimates and no determinations of tensile strength loss rates were made.

Copolyaminotriazole

Schmitt and Polistina [48] have recently shown that a group of polyaminotriazoles are biodegradable film-formers. The

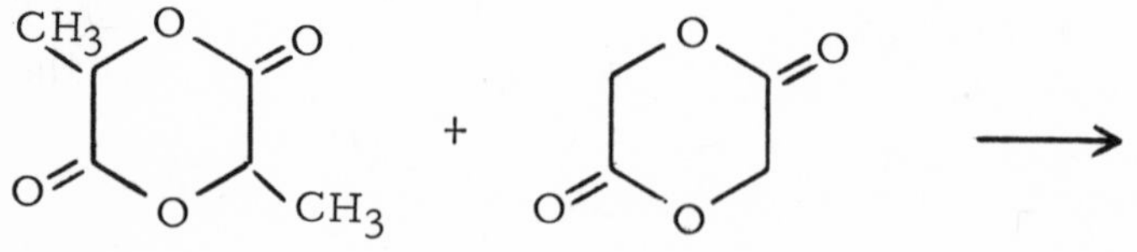

$$---OCHCO_2CHCO - OCH_2CO_2CH_2CO---$$

FIGURE 3. Synthesis of poly(lactide-co-glycolide).

$$H_2NNHCO(CH_2)_nCONHNH_2 \; + \; H_2NNHCO(CH_2)_mCONHNH_2 \longrightarrow$$

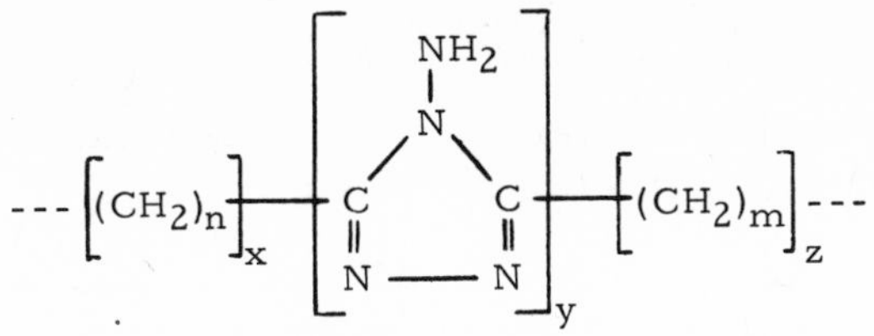

FIGURE 4. Synthesis of polyaminotriazole.

polymers are prepared by condensing acid dihydrazides as shown in Figure 4. Copolymers prepared from a variety of dicarboxylic acid hydrazides were evaluated in rabbits up to 180 days and were found to be biodegradable provided the nitrogen content was between 31.5% and 35.5% by weight.

BIODEGRADABLE NATURAL POLYMERS

Polysaccharide Derivatives

Various polysaccharides have been described as possessing surgical utility although, in general, their strength is not outstanding when compared to other classes of materials.

Bishop [49] reported that fibers useful in surgery could be prepared by extruding the ethyl ether of dextran. Benzyl ethers were also prepared and degrees of substitution of between 1.5 and 3 ether groups per anydroglucose unit appeared to be optimum. Plasticization with phthalate esters was found to be necessary.

Smith [50] showed that, whereas the sodium salts of cellulose acid ethers, for example, sodium carboxymethylcellulose, are not useful as implants, the free acid ethers are suitable after stretching and heat setting. These materials may also be prepared by crosslinking the carboxyl groups with polyvalent metal salts derived from aluminum, chromium or iron. A method for preparing an absorbable base for carrying radioisotopes has been developed utilizing hydroxypropylmethylcellulose [51]. The isotope and

cellulose derivative are combined in a solution which is then converted into easily handled fibers.

Amylose, after being subjected to high temperatures and
pressures, is converted into an extrudable plastic which results
in fibers of relatively low tenacity. Barger and Mumma [52]
claimed that such material is absorbable and useful as sutures
and dressings.

A new class of biodegradable polymers was developed by Kim,
Stannett and Gilbert [24]. Although not directly applicable to
medicine, the principle is of interest. These workers prepared
block copolymers of cellulose triacetate with either diphenylmethane diisocyanate or m-toluene diisocyanate. Terpolymers
were also prepared by adding propylene glycol to this system.
The resulting block copolymers, after deacetylation of the cellulose
component, were labile to attack by cellulase and, in fact, degraded more rapidly than cellulose itself. Although cellulases do
not commonly exist in mammalian tissues, the principle of designing polymers with blocks susceptible to the action of proteases
or other enzymes may be applicable to many problems in this field.

Cellulose itself is not considered a totally biodegradable material, although cotton suture implants do, in fact, lose strength
over extended periods of in vivo residence. However, if regenerated cellulose is oxidized with nitric oxide, a number of the primary hydroxymethyl groups are converted to corresponding carboxyl derivatives [53]. This form of cellulose has found commercial utility as an absorbable hemostatic agent. It possesses relatively poor physical strength and has therefore not found wide
application as a support in reconstructive surgery.

Alginates have also been reported to be biodegradable [54, 55,
56] but few alginate implants have been characterized.

Protein Derivatives

The applications of the most widely used biodegradable proteinaceous surgical implant material, collagen, have been discussed in the preceding report and elsewhere in detail. Gelatin,
a degradation product of collagen, has also found application as an
absorbable agent. For surgical use, gelatin is prepared as a foam
or film and crosslinked with formaldehyde to decrease its solubility.

These materials have little structural wet strength and find utility primarily in hemostasis and in the filling of voids after tissue resection [57].

Since collagen and gelatin are both proteins, they have the potential for inciting immune responses. However, the level of antigenicity is low and related adverse clinical phenomena are rarely reported.

Gerendas [58] has described the preparation of absorbable prosthetic appliances derived from fibrin. The fibrin is obtained from plasma clots and, after purification, is admixed with water and glycerol, and compression-molded at elevated temperatures into various shapes. The devices may be crosslinked with formaldehyde to control the absorption time, reported to be between two weeks and ten months. Myosin, isolated from muscle, may be incorporated to improve the mechanical properties of the resultant devices.

It is apparent that the development of the natural and synthetic biodegradable polymers considered in this discussion has progressed in response to increasingly clearer definitions of needs for materials with special characteristics. For example, exceptionally strong fibers are required for sutures; bulky, perhaps porous masses are indicated for tissue void filling; flexible but rapidly absorbing forms are suitable for drug release vehicles. It is to be expected that the wide variety of polymer systems with varied and special characteristics presently available will allow increasingly successful applications to the many problems in medicine and surgery requiring such materials.

REFERENCES

1.   Salthouse, T. N., Williams, J. A., and Willigan, D. A., Surg., Gynecol., Obstet., 129, 691 (1969).

2.   Nichols, J. and Kronenthal, R. L., Kozarstvi, 13, 380 (1963); Chem. Abs. 60, 10942 (1964).

3.   Chvapil, M., Kronenthal, R. L., and Van Winkle, W., Jr., Int. Rev. Connect. Tissue Res., 6, 1 (1973).

4.   Wade, C. W. R. and Leonard, F., J. Biomed. Mater. Res.,
     6, 215 (1972).

5.   Mattei, F. and Kronenthal, R. L. Unpublished data.

6.   Miyamae, T., Mori, S., and Takeda, Y., assignors to
     Ajinomoto Co., Inc, U. S. Patent 3,371,069 (1968).

7.   Randall, A. A., assignor to Courtaulds Ltd., British Patent
     1,049,290 (1966).

8.   Bamford, C. H., Elliott, A., and Hanby, W. E., Synthetic
     Polypeptides, Academic Press, New York, 1956.

9.   Goodman, M. and Kirshenbaum, G. S., assignors to Sutures,
     Inc., U. S. Patent 3,773,737 (1973).

10. Nachinkin, O. I., Khromova, T. G., and Ulitin, O. N.,
     Khim. Volokna, No. 6, 29-33 (1966); Chem. Abs. 66,
     56444 (1967).

11. Shelton, E. M. and Thompson, W. L., assignors to
     Johnson & Johnson, U. S. Patent 2,447,140 (1948).

12. Herrmann, W. O., Hammer, F., Kassel, B., and Hachnel,
     W., assignors to Chemische Forschungsgesellschaft mbH,
     U. S. Patent 2,092,512 (1937).

13. Middendorf, L., Med. Chem., 4, 573 (1942); Chem. Abs.
     38, 5367 (1944).

14. Dayer, J. M., Fischer, A., Besson, A., and Mirkovitch,
     V., Helv. Chir. Acta, 36, 296 (1969).

15. Fritsch, S., Pharmazie, 22, 41 (1967).

16. Marans, N. S., assignor to W. R. Grace & Co., U. S.
     Patent 3,111,469 (1963).

17. Baptist, J. N., assignor to W. R. Grace & Co., U. S.
     Patents 3,036,959 (1962), 3,044,942 (1962), and 3,225,766
     (1965).

18.   Kronenthal, R. L.   Unpublished data.

19.   Frazza, E. J. and Schmitt, E. E., J. Biomed. Mater.
      Res., Symp. No. 1, 43 (1971).

20.   Wykoff, T. W., Laryngoscope, 83, 1072 (1973).

21.   Schmitt, E. E. and Polistina, R. A., assignors to
      American Cyanamid Co., U. S. Patents 3,463,158 (1969),
      3,620,218 (1971), and 3,739,773 (1973).

22.   Semp, B. A., assignor to American Cyanamid Co., U. S.
      Patent 3,810,458 (1974).

23.   Schmitt, E. E., Suen, T. J., and Updegraff, I. H.,
      assignors to American Cyanamid Co., U. S. Patent
      3,784,585 (1974).

24.   Kim, S., Stannett, V. T., and Gilbert, R. D., J. Polym.
      Sci., Polym. Lett. Ed., 11, 731 (1973).

25.   Dittrich, W. and Schulz, R. C., Angew. Makromol. Chem.,
      15, 109 (1971).

26.   Higgins, N. A., assignor to E. I. du Pont de Nemours &
      Co., U. S. Patent 2,676,945 (1954).

27.   Daicell Ltd., Japanese Patent 347/70; Chem. Abs. 72,
      101248 (1970).

28.   Tonelli, A. E. and Flory, P. J., Macromolecules, 2, 225
      (1969).

29.   Brant, D. A., Tonelli, A. E., and Flory, P. J.,
      Macromolecules, 2, 228 (1969).

30.   Mhala, M. M. and Mishra, J. P., Indian J. Chem., 8, 243
      (1970).

31.   Kulkarni, R. K., Pani, K. C., Neuman, C., and Leonard,
      F., Arch. Surg., 93, 839 (1966).

32. Kulkarni, R. K., Moore, E. G., Hegyeli, A. F., and
     Leonard, F., J. Biomed. Mater. Res., 5, 169 (1971).

33. Hodge, J. W., Jr., Dimensional Stability of Poly(D, L-
     Lactic Acid) Monofilament, U. S. Nat. Tech. Inform.
     Serv., AD Rept. No. 742,719, 1971.

34. Fouty, R. A., assignor to Ethicon, Inc., Canadian Patents
     808,731 (1969) and 923,245 (1973).

35. Schneider, A. K., assignor to Ethicon, Inc., U. S. Patent
     3,636,956 (1972).

36. Schneider, A. K., assignor to Ethicon, Inc., U. S. Patent
     3,797,499 (1974).

37. Thomas, P. A., Experimental Evaluation of Woven Poly-
     lactic Acid, Polyester Tubes as Tracheal Prostheses, U. S.
     Nat. Tech. Inform. Serv., AD Rept. No. 767,305, 1973.

38. Getter, L., Cutright, D. E., Bhaskar, S. N., and Augsburg,
     J. K., J. Oral Surg., 30, 344 (1972).

39. Cutright, D. E. and Hunsuck, E. E., Oral Surg., Oral Med.,
     Oral Pathol., 33, 28 (1972).

40. Cutright, D. E., Beasley, J. D., III, and Perez, B., ibid.,
     32, 165 (1971).

41. Gregory, J. B., Schwope, A. D., and Wise, D. L.,
     Development of a Synthetic Polymer Burn Coating, U. S.
     Nat. Tech. Inform. Serv., AD Rept. No. 759,381, 1973.

42. Brady, J. M., Cutright, D. E., Miller, R. A., Battistone,
     G. C., and Hunsuck, E. E., J. Biomed. Mater. Res., 7,
     155 (1973).

43. Hegyeli, A. F., ibid., 7, 205 (1973).

44. Jackanicz, T. M., Nash, H. A., Wise, D. L., and Gregory,
     J. B., Contraception, 8, 227 (1973).

45.   Boswell, G. A., Jr. and Scribner, R. M., assignors to
       E. I. du Pont de Nemours & Co., U. S. Patent 3,773,919
       (1973).

46.   Wasserman, D. and Levy, A., assignors to Ethicon, Inc.,
       Canadian Patent 950,308 (1974).

47.   Cutright, D. E., Perez, B., Beasley, J. D., III, Larson,
       W. J., and Posey, W. R., Oral Surg., Oral Med., Oral
       Pathol., 37, 142 (1974).

48.   Schmitt, E. E. and Polistina, R. A., assignors to
       American Cyanamid Co., U. S. Patent 3,809,683 (1974).

49.   Bishop, A. E., assignor to The Commonwealth Engineering
       Co. of Ohio, U. S. Patent 2,914,415 (1959).

50.   Smith, D. F., U. S. Patent 3,757,786 (1973).

51.   Institut Meditsinskoi Radiologii AMN, SSR, German Patent
       2,011,612 (1974).

52.   Barger, J. W. and Mumma, C. E., assignors to U. S.
       Dept. Economic Development, German Patent 2,001,533
       (1971).

53.   Ashton, W. H. and Moser, C. E., assignors to Johnson &
       Johnson, U. S. Patent 3,364,200 (1968).

54.   Lubet-Moncla, Z. L., French Patent 1,452,012 (1966).

55.   Bonniksen, C. W., British Patent 653,341 (1951).

56.   Skelton, L. Z. and Graham, J., assignors to Medical
       Alginates Ltd., British Patent 882,565 (1961).

57.   Tucker, H. A., Absorbable Gelatin (Gelfoam) Sponge,
       Charles C. Thomas, Springfield, Ill., 1965.

58.   Gerendas, M., U. S. Patent 3,523,807 (1970).

BLOOD COMPATIBILITY OF SYNTHETIC POLYMERS:

PERSPECTIVE AND PROBLEMS

R. E. Baier

Chemical Sciences Section, Calspan, Inc.,
4455 Genesee Street, Buffalo, New York 14221

INTRODUCTION

This brief narrative presents the understanding which I believe has been achieved among workers in the field of blood compatibility of nonphysiologic materials. The key problem area remaining to be clarified is that of protein adsorption and its influence on subsequent cell adhesive events. Figure 1 charts the general interactions which occur when blood contacts foreign solid surfaces. It had been thought until the late 1960s that protein adsorption on the solid surface, ultimately leading to blood gelation by pathways involving the numbered coagulation factors (XII, XIII, etc.) was independent of the parallel events of platelet adhesion to the same solid. Initial platelet adhesion to the bare foreign surface, followed by platelet aggregation into the blood stream, was presumed to mimic the kinetic and thermodynamic events observed in platelet aggregation studies in the absence of foreign solid surface contact, ultimately leading to the formation of a white thrombus mass.

We have since shown, and have been universally supported in this finding by other workers, that platelets do not, and perhaps cannot, adhere to nonphysiologic substrates without a preconditioning layer of adsorbed protein. That layer of adsorbed protein is, at least through the normal time delay prior to the adhesion of platelets to any foreign solid surface (between 30 seconds and one minute, depending upon the flow situation), certainly dominated by

139

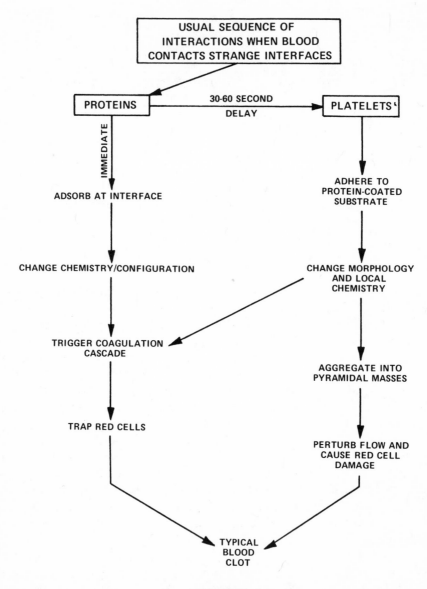

FIGURE 1

fibrinogen. It should be immediately noted that this preconditioning film builds by spontaneous adsorption, in the presence of potentially adhesive cells such as platelets, in a time much too short to be identified with protein films studied after adsorption equilibrium has been achieved. Equilibrium protein adsorption is a process which takes at least many minutes at normal physiological protein concentrations and even hours and days, as reported in some model experiments. Thus, experiments which attempt to deduce the composition and configuration of adsorbed protein films after adsorption-desorption equilibrium has been achieved, although interesting and important physicochemically, are essentially irrelevant to the problems of blood compatibility and cell adhesion to synthetic material surfaces in the overwhelming majority of biological circumstances.

COMPETING CONCEPTS OF PROTEIN ADSORPTION

It is most important to inquire into the specifics of the adsorption process in the early period after first contact of whole blood or any other biological macromolecule- and cell-containing solution with strange interfaces. Two models for the adsorption of macromolecules, and particularly biological macromolecules such as proteins at solid-liquid interfaces are prevalent. Figures 2, 3, and 4 show on the left and right sides, respectively, the sequence of events proposed in each model. The sequence of steps illustrated in the left scheme is considered the more radical picture today, although it was the historically accepted model until careful studies of the adsorption of nonbiological random-tangle-configured macromolecules, such as polystyrene in special solvents, were widely reported over the past two decades. The right side picture is the now more widely accepted sequence of events in concordance with modern polymer theory. The left picture with deeper historical roots is today most vigorously defended by Nyilas and colleagues*, who focus their experimental program on microcalorimetric analyses of the details of protein adsorption on foreign solid substrates [1]. The right side model is today most consistent with the interpretation of the polymer interface group led by Stromberg at the National Bureau of Standards*, who focus their experimental program on ellipsometric and infrared spectroscopic analyses of protein adsorption events at foreign solid surfaces [2]. I find the left model more intuitively satisfying and the

_____

*Supported financially by the NHLI

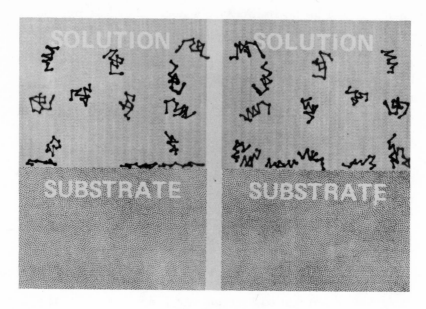

FIGURE 2

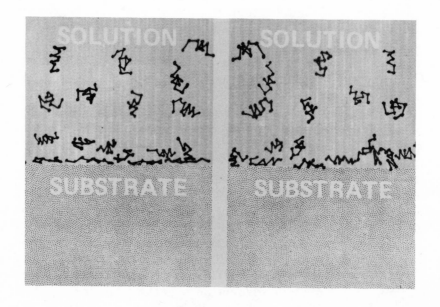

FIGURE 3

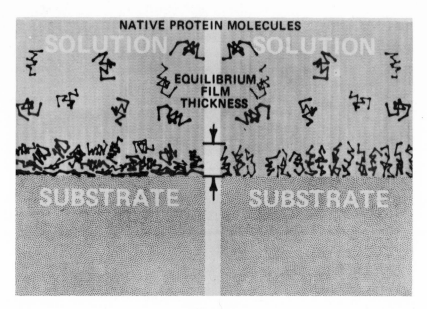

FIGURE 4

work by microcalorimetry more convincing than that currently
coming from the Bureau of Standards and from a host of other
laboratories reaching the same general conclusions. Note, from
Figure 2, that the left model assumes the initially arriving macromolecules which, in the situation under discussion here are blood
proteins, to accommodate themselves to the solid-liquid interface
in a way which takes maximum advantage of the surface area available. This leads to potentially large and essentially irreversible
changes in protein configuration and binding at the substrate. The
right side model suggests that, although the initially arriving
macromolecules may accommodate themselves to the entire surface area available, they do so in a less irreversible way and can
potentially resume their essentially native (that is, solution state)
configuration. As Figure 3 illustrates, later on in time, and in
the case of blood, certainly less than 30 seconds after first contact, the left side model for protein adsorption depicts secondary
layers of less configurationally distorted macromolecules adsorbing to, or partially between, the original population (considered
the monolayer) of surface localized molecules. The right model
depicts subsequently arriving macromolecules as competing with
the originally adsorbed matter for sites at the interface, and all
such interfacially localized components as being in essentially the

same configuration and bound with equal strength. Figure 4 suggests the situation found at equilibrium, and it is most important
to note that it never seems to be achieved in those areas where
cells adhere irreversibly in the two models, as will be discussed
later. In the left model, at the attainment of adsorption-desorption equilibrium, the originally deposited monolayer remains as
deposited. Monolayer is considered in the most classical interpretation of this term as representing macromolecules having deformed themselves into their most extended achievable planar
configurations - a convenient fiction since steric hindrance, H-
bonding, fixed bond angles, and covalent intrachain links such as
disulfide bonds resist this "unfolding". On top of this originally
adsorbed population of effectively irreversibly bound components
are a succession of less and less configurationally distorted and
less strongly bound components in an unspecified number of layers,
until the outermost film aspect is, in fact, in equilibrium with the
solution phase molecules and exhibits essentially native protein
properties. In the right hand model, another definition of monolayer is invoked, and it too has its historical roots; here, only a
single layer of adsorbed macromolecules is present, and these
are in the same essentially native configuration, all equally available for spontaneous desorption under the right conditions, and
also exhibiting primarily solution state protein properties under
equilibrium conditions. It is the achievement in both models of an
essentially native outermost layer of matter that eliminates the
thermodynamic gradient or "strangeness" at the interface, and
limits the continued avalanche of material from the solution to the
surface localized state.

Proponents of these two models, in numerous formal and in-
formal debates over the past few years, have been able to adjust
their pictures so that both the growing and the equilibrium films,
reached by either the left or right side route, would have the same
thickness and refractive index, and the same fraction of surface
bound groups when averaged over the total mass of material adsorbed, at the same times. Both models predict ultimate adsorption-desorption equilibrium with native molecules in solution.
This has caused experimental difficulties in defining which of the
two routes is in fact followed in the pattern of protein adsorption
preceding platelet adhesion and thrombus generation on synthetic
materials such as the common polymers of modern commerce.

ATTACHMENT OF THE FIRST LAYER OF PLATELETS

It is most important to distinguish between these models, even though during the course of building to equilibrium thickness, the adsorbing films of each model can have the same average thickness and surface bound fractions at the same times, since they predict different surface chemistries until adsorption equilibrium is finally achieved. Studies of the kinetics of platelet adhesion to foreign solid surfaces in fresh flowing blood, i.e., not chemically modified or anticoagulated, consistently verified in fluid flow and microcinematographic experiments in a number of laboratories, make it clear that the platelets adhere during the course of film buildup and not after equilibrium film thicknesses have been achieved [3, 4]. It is timely, therefore, to evaluate likely explanations for this mandatory "conditioning" film buildup to a peculiar thickness and/or configuration and/or chemical and/or electronic array prior to cell adhesion. At this point, it is useful to recall that groups at McMaster University and at the University of Toronto have shown that platelets will adhere neither to normally intact fibrinogen nor to completely formed fibrin, but rather only to polymerizing fibrinogen [5, 6]. This provides a clue to the events occurring in the initially adsorbed layers of fibrinogen, which antibody studies show to dominate the earliest adsorbed layers formed on foreign solid substrates in blood. The analogy to wet paint is instructive; fly specks adhere neither to liquid paint nor to the fully cured paint which coats a house, but while the paint film is still wet, after having recently been applied, it is exceptionally receptive to arriving solid matter and tends to anchor it there permanently. The analogy is imperfect, of course, and should be considered no more than a popularization of the events described. In fact, it is a subject of most serious concern to those studying events of cell adhesion, and especially platelet adhesion at nonphysiologic interfaces, to learn the true reasons for the 30 seconds to one minute lag time before cells become adherent to solid substrates, and then do so only through the medium of an intervening proteinaceous film.

It is also instructive to recall at this time, that both simplified fluid mechanical considerations and electrostatic-electrodynamic considerations predict the nearly absolute exclusion of the normally discoid-shaped platelets from the foreign solid surfaces over which blood flows [7, 8]. In order to overcome both the fluid flow restrictions and electrostatic repulsions keeping the disc-shaped cells from essentially flat foreign surfaces, it is necessary

to invoke modifications in the cell surface architecture to incorporate probes of extremely low radii of curvature. These probes
are the spikes, microvilli or pseudopods about which an enormous
body of technical literature, seeking an explanation for their role
and mode of formation, has been generated. An alternative suggestion inspired by the work of Blackshear and co-workers [9] is that
the material of the spontaneously adsorbed proteinaceous films may
be serving, in a nonspecific manner, as the equivalent of numerous
probes of exceptionally low radius of curvature which bridge the
gap between normally-shaped cells and the substrate without difficulty; fluid mechanics and common colloid theories predict that
a gap must always exist [10]. Using language introduced by
Blackshear, with respect to red cell adhesion to foreign surfaces,
we might consider the initially adsorbed proteinaceous strands as
microtethers which provide the first bridging links between solid
synthetic polymers or other foreign substrates and the arriving
cells. Such an explanation is consistent with recent experiments
and theory with respect to cell adhesion in other circumstances,
as presented by Maroudas [11]. It also redeems the notion of
direct molecule-to-molecule contact being responsible for adhesive events in biology without requiring the secondary minimum
argument which many theorists have labored over in an attempt to
explain the normal gap existing between individual cells in tissue
ensembles [12].

INITIAL EVENTS AT BOTH THROMBOGENIC
AND THROMBORESISTANT INTERFACES

Returning to the details of protein adsorption on foreign solid
surfaces, it is important to recognize the differences existing
among materials exposed to protein solutions and which can be
demonstrated even in the nature of the equilibrium adsorbed films
formed. The group at the Bureau of Standards has reported, for
example, that the blood proteins fibrinogen, prothrombin and
serum albumin, adsorbed to surfaces of varying surface-free energies, with each protein giving about the same amount adsorbed on
varying substrates, will have, on the lower energy substrates, an
extension of the absorbed matter out into the solution phase significantly greater than that from the higher energy substrates [2].
The implication is that proteins adsorbed to foreign solid substrates
will be less configurationally distorted on the lower energy surfaces. I have argued elsewhere that such correlations can be taken
only so far, and that the exceptionally low energy surfaces such as

the fluorocarbon polymers, because of the complexity and variety
of monomeric units within proteins, will bind those biological
macromolecules in a more configurationally distorted manner than
will some of the moderately low surface energy materials [13, 14].
I continue to hold that minimum protein distortion may ultimately
be experimentally associated with maximum protein extension
(maximum retention of native structure) out into the solution medium, and that this condition will exist for a narrow midrange of
surface free energies. For example, if one ranks the surface free
energies of polymers according to the empirical parameter of
critical surface tension determined for each in air, the most biocompatible range seems to be between 20 and 30 dynes/cm.
Nyilas [15] has independently endorsed this suggestion that minimum protein distortion in the initially adsorbed film will correlate with maximum blood compatibility and has introduced the
phrase "low interaction energies ensure short residence times".

Most of the testing of nonphysiologic materials for blood compatibility has relied upon reasonably direct methods, such as the
insertion of representative polymers as small cylindrical rings
into the canine inferior vena cava for periods of two hours in an
acute test, or two weeks in a chronic test. Gott, et al. [16] showed
that most such rings become fully blocked with blood clots at the
end of only two hours so that the sequence of events which has
initiated this disastrous consequence is totally masked from the
analyst. We have subsequently shown that simple stripping of such
clots from the lumen of vena cava rings always leads to cohesive
failure within the red cell-fibrin mesh near, but not at the interface [17]. Thus, the sequence of early events cannot be recon-
structed from an after-the-fact or reverse analysis with respect
to the originally attached platelet + protein lamella. The techni-
cally very difficult experiments which attempt to visualize and
carefully analyze the initial events at fresh blood-foreign solid
interfaces, such as those we reported six years ago with Dutton
and co-workers [3, 18, 19], assume ever greater importance.
In those experiments, well documented by color microcinematog-
raphy, axial blood from the transected jugular vein of lightly anesthetized canines was allowed, after displacing a physiologic saline
buffer, to impinge on the face of various test materials in a stag-
nation point chamber such as that developed and still used by
Petschek and co-workers [4]. Epoxy slabs were used as the test
substrates, the experiments were stopped by flushing with a fixa-
tive solution at various times from only a few seconds to about ten
minutes following the first blood contact, and the test surfaces

were subsequently postfixed with osmium tetroxide, embedded in
more epoxy, cross-sectioned with a microtome, and finally post-
stained before observation in a transmission electron microscope.
Information was gathered as to the nature and sequence of the
earliest events occurring at these interfaces even when those
events were at the single macromolecular monolayer level.

After a few seconds of blood contact, a very thin heavy metal
staining film, known to be proteinaceous from ancillary experiments by internal reflection infrared spectroscopy, was present.
At the end of about one minute of blood contact with the surface, a
granular layer of dimensions between 50 and 200 Å could be seen
uniformly coating the surface. At this time, no specific distin-
guishable characteristics, such as periodicity along fine fibers or
globular regions, which might indicate the presence of one or another of the specific blood proteins, could be found. By this time
however, in the majority of regions observed, an original layer
of singly deposited platelets was already present and beginning to
show morphological changes, particularly pseudopod formation
and evidence of degranulation. The number density of platelets
found in such experiments was always in the range of about 70-100
platelets per 1,000 square microns, as quantitated by Friedman
and co-workers [20] and substantiated by others. The reason for
the lack of complete surface coverage by the arriving platelets is
a subject of continuing speculation. Again considering the fluid
mechanical arguments and electrostatic repulsion arguments which
have been adduced to explain why normally shaped platelets cannot
reach the foreign solid substrate closely enough to adhere in the
first place, we might invoke similar arguments in explaining why
the zone between the small platelet hillocks might be similarly
forbidden to subsequently arriving cells. Those subsequently arriving cells should have an enhanced likelihood of colliding with
and, if the cell surface adhesive factors are also activated, aggre-
gating with the originally adherent cells.

SECONDARY EVENTS AT THROMBOGENIC INTERFACES

No matter what final mechanism is accepted, it is clear that
in the regions between the initially adherent cells, including subsequently adherent platelets and white cells, predominately segmented neutrophils, the originally adsorbed protein film is not a
static layer. Vroman and co-workers [21] have demonstrated
that, from a period of about 30 seconds to one minute, such films

are chemically converted or configurationally modified in such manner that they are no longer recognizable by fibrinogen-antibody or adhesive to arriving platelets. Our own electron micrographs reveal that the film thickens to about 800 Å, becomes more fuzzy in appearance, and frank strands and masses of fibrin as identified from the known electron microscopic periodicity of fibrin in those few instances when such periodicity has been noted emanate out into the lumen from this film. It is the sequence of events in these cell-free areas which is best identified with the blood coagulation scheme earlier introduced and understood to involve the numbered blood coagulation factors. In the overwhelming majority of cases, the originally adsorbed proteinaceous film supports platelet adhesion in the most damaging sense; those platelets are essentially permanently adherent, undergo extreme morphological changes, and are most attractive to their subsequently arriving neighbors with which they aggregate into three-dimensional pyramidal masses. Such thrombus collections extend into the blood volume where they secondarily disturb flow patterns and assist in the avalanche of coagulation factors, fibrin formation and the mechanical trapping and involvement of the larger red cells which are even more rigidly excluded from the interfacial zone by fluid mechanical effects [7].

In seeking to characterize the initially adsorbed protein film which supports this secondary sequence of adverse events, we have attempted to use contact angle measurements to deduce a parameter called the critical surface tension. Our previous reports have identified a critical surface tension range in the mid-to-high 30s dynes/cm as characterizing these normally thrombogenic precursor layers. Figure 5B illustrates an embryonic thrombus consisting of only a few platelets adhering to such an adsorbed film whose thickness is about 200 Å. Higher magnification electron micrographs, such as Figure 5A, reveal that the platelet membrane itself is always separated from the foreign solid substrate not only by this adsorbed layer of originally adsorbed proteins but also by a fine fibrous layer of (supposed) protein which seems to be an extracellular coating on the platelet exterior. Booyse and co-workers [22] suggest that this is the platelet surface contractile protein complex which bears striking similarities to the actomyosin complex of smooth and striated muscle and which may be responsible for the original adhesive properties of the cell.

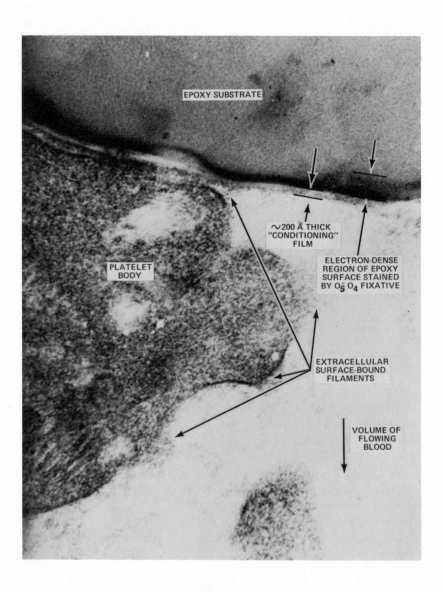

FIGURE 5A

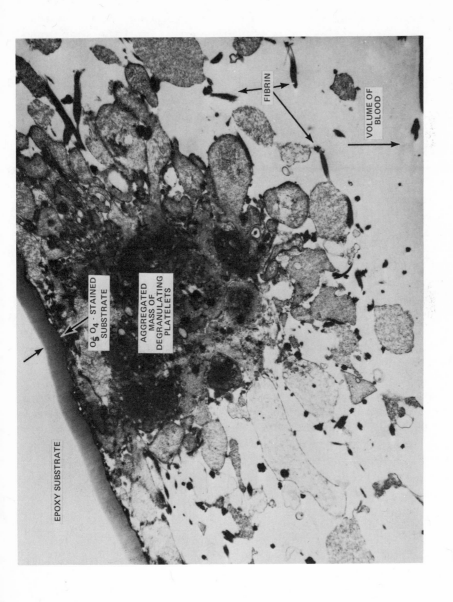

FIGURE 5B

SECONDARY EVENTS AT THROMBO-
RESISTANT INTERFACES

Returning to a consideration of the differences which various
substrates produce on the process of blood gelation and particularly thrombus formation, it is instructive to recall the scanning
electron microscopy done by Schoen [23] on the original layer of
adherent platelets covering the impeller surfaces of blood pumps.
Such scanning electron micrographs show that the platelets originally adherent to the ultimately more thrombogenic substrates
such as metals are flattened, have numerous pseudopods and are
essentially permanently attached. The platelets adherent to the
ultimately thromboresistant surfaces such as pyrolytic carbon and
various polyurethanes maintain their rounded or discoid configurations, and when inspected at later times, have been detached by
either shear forces or through not yet understood mechanisms of
secondary adhesion and scavenging by white cells. It is important
to note, as numerous investigators have since confirmed, that
even well heparinized surfaces do not escape free of adherent
platelets in the early stages, and that these initially adherent
platelets are also morphologically distorted. It is only after erosion of the labile surface coating of heparin begins that the original
layer of platelets is shed and the surface remains, for a reasonably long time, apparently thromboresistant, but not truly so, because of the anticoagulant effects of the high concentration of heparin in the boundary layer adjacent to the test specimen. Thus,
although many workers have confirmed that, independent of the
nature of a significant variety of materials and certainly of almost
all common plastics, all surfaces accumulate the same number
density of platelets over the same time period in well designed
flow experiments, it is no longer reasonable to assume that these
platelets have the same morphological disposition and the same
permanency of attachment to the substrate or stickiness to their
subsequently arriving neighbors.

TRANSITION TO LONG-TERM
BLOOD CONTACT EVENTS

Most workers now agree that the first significant event at
foreign solid surfaces exposed in blood is monomeric fibrinogen
adsorption and distortion. Where these monomers are distorted
or partially aggregated to a sufficient degree, and when thickened
to a sufficient distance from the original substrate, platelets which

are known to be arriving in sufficient number from the initiation
of blood flow but are nonadhering, do actually adhere in a random,
incompletely packed, two -dimensional pattern. This does not
prevent the continuation of protein adsorption, conversion, and
subsequent involvement of Hageman Factor (Factor XII), its distortion and interaction with Factor XI, and subsequent coagulation
events in other areas. The combination of protein coagulation and
gross cell trapping resulting from this secondary process is referred to as blood clotting outside the biomaterials research community. Once such clotting occurs, the events immediately at or
adjacent to the foreign solid-blood interface are so completely ob-
scured by the mass of debris which has attached thereto that attempts to reconstruct the "scene of the crime" have been useless
so far. It is known that the platelet thrombi grow in a pyramidal
shape out into the flowing blood stream in essentially pure cellular
aggregates; it is only after they have grown to a significant thickness of at least a few microns, generally in a wake or teardrop
pattern oriented with the blunt edge upstream, that an interaggre-
gate mesh of fibrin and red cells forms. The ultimate result at
the end of a two-hour implantation period in a Gott ring test, for
example, is a complete lumen-blocking red clot.

Some materials do repeatedly and, therefore, now predictably
persist for not only two hours free of clot in a Gott vena cava ring
test but also for as long as two weeks. It is known that their surfaces support the same initial two events, protein adsorption and
platelet adhesion, as the ultimate clot producing materials. Simple
light microscopic inspections of the thrombogenic and thromboresistant surfaces do not reveal significant differences over a
period of about ten minutes of blood contact. In the thromboresistant specimens, electron microscopic inspection shows that from
times of about ten minutes or more, the originally adherent layer
of morphologically undisturbed platelets which have not become
sticky to their subsequently arriving siblings are surrounded by
white cells. In a process perhaps akin to the phagocytic process
for which these white cells have been specialized by evolution,
platelets are removed from the surface. The solid substrate-
blood interface then continues to experience adsorption and re-
modeling of its proteinaceous coating until a passivating film exists
in long-term and perhaps permanent equilibrium or pseudoequilib-
rium with the flowing blood stream. Characteristics of this passivating film which have been identified to date include its easy
lability or exchangeability into salt solutions or even distilled water, its remarkable monodispersity when studied by exceptionally

sensitive infrared analytical techniques, its low critical surface
tension of 20-30 dynes/cm when challenged by water-immiscible
dispersion-force-only wetting liquids, and high penetrability by
water and water-immiscible or hydrogen-bonding liquids. So far,
the amount of this passivating material which we have been able
to harvest has been subminimal for such other analytical procedures as immunochemistry, ultracentrifugation, optical rotatory
dispersion, or Raman spectroscopy. UV transmission spectroscopy has shown only that it is essentially a pure protein or glycoprotein. In all those cases when, after two hours of inferior vena
cava implantation, a polymeric material has been found to be free
of electron microscopically visible cellular debris, the lumen of
the implanted ring has been coated with enough of this essentially
pure passivating protein to completely mask the underlying polymeric chemistry by both spectral and wettability criteria. Even
heparinized specimens which have subsequently shed their adherent platelets continue to hold a layer of protein to their surface,
although such protein must be continuously renewed since these
surfaces are constantly eroding at a slow rate.

RELATED INVESTIGATIONS AND SPECULATIONS

With respect to the characterization of the passivated surface, it has always been found in our laboratory that polymeric
and inorganic substrates with high critical surface tension will
acquire, within a two-hour thrombus-free implantation, a critical
surface tension of about 25-30 dynes/cm, as judged by water-
immiscible, nonhydrogen-bonding test liquids. One of the most
impressive of the early materials examined was not polymeric in
the traditional sense: pyrolytic carbon. This material, polished
with one-quarter micron diamond and rendered organic-free before
implantation, has a critical surface tension near 50 dynes/cm,
but after both two hours and two weeks of thrombus-free implantation in the canine inferior vena cava, has a marvelously monodisperse energy-lowering coating of glycoprotein which has yet to
be further analyzed since it has only been present in such exceedingly small quantities in experiments carried out to date. This
protein has extraordinary surface activity in the sense that it will
depress the surface tension of aqueous solutions by some 30 or
more dynes/cm, and will show, with water-immiscible diagnostic
liquids, a nonwetting behavior extrapolating to an apparent critical
surface tension in the high 20 dynes/cm. In an attempt to understand the interaction of such a film with the continuously arriving

platelets, we have now begun a series of preliminary studies of the
surface chemistry of the platelet periphery as well. Here we
enter an area of considerable controversy, in that the surfaces of
living cells can exhibit a very high apparent surface-free energy
when tested with aqueous or other hydrogen bond-capable fluids and
simultaneously a quite low surface free energy when probed with
nonpolar organic or van der Waals' force-only-capable liquids.
It becomes a matter for both future conjecture and experimentation
to examine the role of water as bound and structured in, at, and
around the proteinaceous layers at both the adsorbed film and cell
periphery, and to decide whether or not the forces of recognition
or interaction between cells and surfaces, and subsequently cells
and cells, are manifested by the high surface energy suite of polar
and hydrogen bonding interactions or are more fundamentally related to the universal dispersion force interactions. In the latter
case, one would have to consider the heretical notion that water
might act in biological contact phenomena, especially cell-surface
interactions, as a universal ether of sorts which could be practically, if not theoretically, ignored.

There are many other current relevant investigations which
have not been discussed in the foregoing paragraphs. Some should
be mentioned here, because they emphasize the specifics of protein adsorption as related to subsequent cell adhesion. It is ironic
in a way that our earlier publications were almost wholly devoted
to the then disagreeable notion that proteins at nonphysiologic
interfaces could maintain some degree of their native structural
integrity, as against the now four-decade-old thesis that all proteins at all nonphysiologic interfaces completely distort to the ex-
tended-chain β structure form in which no biological specificity
could be expected [24, 25, 26]. I now find myself vigorously defending the prospect that proteins spontaneously adsorbed at nonphysiologic interfaces do lose some of their native structure, and
thus modify their function and specificity, against challenges of
the polymer interface community. Nevertheless, I continue to
favor the left side model for the route to equilibrium adsorption
as illustrated in Figures 2, 3, and 4.

Along these lines, let us consider the demonstrably useful
technique of precoating biomedical device surfaces with the only
blood protein which is not claimed to be a glycoprotein, albumin.
A significant amount of evidence has been accumulated about the
ability of albumin to remain more native than most other molecules

at nonphysiologic interfaces and therefore exhibit better equilibrium with its solution phase. Albumin treatment can usefully extend the thrombus-free time of blood contacting materials in extracorporeal circuits. I propose that the easy exchangeability of albumin into the flowing blood volume, after having been forcefully built to its equilibrium thickness by the precoating procedure, underlies this significant extension of useful time of some materials in contact with blood. Unfortunately, such precoating procedures must fail when the adsorption-desorption equilibrium can no longer be maintained, and the population of molecules at the interface changes to a more adverse mixture.

With respect to the hypothesis briefly noted here that a peculiar range of critical surface tension characterizes materials with the greatest likelihood of biocompatibility through the mechanism of minimizing the configurational changes in the proteins which all surfaces inevitably adsorb, it is pertinent to note the recent results of Kolobow and co-workers [27] that polydimethylsiloxane, when free of silica and having a critical surface tension in the range of 20-30 dynes/cm, shows significant extension of its thrombus-free blood contact time. Thus, by having solved a surface texture problem first, and probably a surface chemical problem of trace exposure of foreign silica particles as well, a significant improvement has been made in the already useful class of silicone polymers. There are numerous other materials, including the segmented polyurethane elastomer known as Biomer*, and long alkyl side chain substituted polymers of a variety of backbone types [28], which also exhibit a properly low, but not extremely low, critical surface tension and may have significant promise of long-term blood compatibility.

There is also recent evidence that, except for the requirements to keep blood moving at some rate, flow perturbations may have been overemphasized as a cause of blood clotting and thrombus formation in the past. Ward and co-workers [29], at the University of Toronto, have shown for example, that surface texturally rough silicone rubber which normally has a high incidence of platelet adhesion, aggregation and ultimate thrombogenesis, can be significantly improved in its contact relation with blood by simply outgassing the entrapped air from the microcrevices and the surface textural inhomogeneities prior to blood contact. This

---

*Ethicon, Inc., Somerville, N. J.

work clearly suggests that remnant pockets of potentially renewable air-liquid interface may be responsible for the denaturing event which forms the first nidus for platelet adhesion and ultimate thrombogenesis on these otherwise proper (surface chemical) substrates. Thus, it is not a flow irregularity which has rendered such surfaces blood-incompatible in the past, but another surface chemical problem which had not been properly recognized.

Finally, defending the neglect of surface charge in the foregoing discussion, recall that surface charge manipulations of biomedical materials have not been successful to date and continue to be difficult to achieve without secondary damage to the blood elements. Most synthetic polyelectrolytes bearing the net negative charges that some workers suggest are desirable, for example, must be inserted into the blood stream as neutralized specimens. The neutralizing cations modify in the extreme the local blood pH, causing numerous secondary complications not originally anticipated. When such synthetic polyelectrolytes have been fabricated and implanted, the ultimate results have not been promising; all such implants generally form complete thrombi and lumen-blocking clots well before the two-week period which is considered the criterion of significant thromboresistance in the inferior vena cava.

REFERENCES

1. Nyilas, E., Chiu, T. H., Herzlinger, G. A., and Federico, A., Microcalorimetric Study of the Interaction of Plasma Proteins with Synthetic Surfaces, Annual Report on Contract NIH-NOL-HB-3-2917, 1974, U. S. Nat. Tech. Inform. Serv., Springfield, Va.

2. Fenstermaker, C. A., Grant, W. H., Morrissey, B. W., Smith, L. E., and Stromberg, R. R., Interaction of Plasma Proteins with Surfaces, U. S. Nat. Tech. Inform. Serv., Springfield, Va., Rept. No. NBSIR 74-470, 1974.

3. Dutton, R. C., Baier, R. E., Dedrick, R. L., and Bowman, R. L., Trans. Amer. Soc. Artif. Intern. Organs, 14, 57 (1968).

4. Madras, P. N., Morton, W. A., and Petschek, H. E., Fed. Proc., Fed. Amer. Soc. Exp. Biol., 30, 1665 (1971).

5.   Niewiarowski, S., Regoeczi, E., and Mustard, J. F., Ann.
     N. Y. Acad. Sci., 201, 72 (1972).

6.   Mustard, J. F., Glynn, M. F., Nishizawa, E. E., and
     Packham, M. A., Fed. Proc., Fed. Amer. Soc. Exp. Biol.,
     26, 106 (1967).

7.   Brenner, H. and Bungay, P. M., ibid., 30, 1565 (1971).

8.   Weiss, L., ibid., 30, 1649 (1971).

9.   Blackshear, P. L., Jr., Forstrom, R. J., Dorman, F. D.,
     and Voss, G. O., ibid., 30, 1600 (1971).

10. Parsegian, V. A., Ann. Rev. Biophys. Bioeng., 2, 221
     (1973).

11. Maroudas, N. G., J. Theor. Biol., 1974 (in press).

12. Weiss, L., in The Cell Periphery, Metastasis, and Other
     Contact Phenomena, A. Neuberger and E. L. Tatum, Eds.,
     Frontiers of Biology, 7, (1968).

13. Baier, R. E., in Adhesion in Biological Systems, R. S.
     Manly, Ed., Academic Press, New York, 1970.

14. Baier, R. E., Bull. N. Y. Acad. Med., 48, 257 (1972).

15. Nyilas, E., personal communication.

16. Gott, V. L. and Furuse, A., Fed. Proc., Fed. Amer. Soc.
     Exp. Biol., 30, 1679 (1971).

17. DePalma, V. A., Baier, R. E., Ford, J. W., Gott, V. L.,
     and Furuse, A., in Biomaterials for Skeletal and Cardio-
     vascular Applications, C. Homsy and C. D. Armediades,
     Eds., Interscience Publishers, John Wiley and Sons,
     New York, 1972.

18. Dutton, R. C., Webber, A. J., Johnson, S. A., and Baier,
     R. E., J. Biomed. Mater. Res., 3, 13 (1969).

19. Baier, R. E., and Dutton, R. C., ibid., 3, 191 (1969).

20.   Friedman, L. I., Liem, H., Grabowski, E. F., Leonard,
      E. F., and McCord, C. W., Trans. Amer. Soc. Artif.
      Intern. Organs, 16, 63 (1970).

21.   Vroman, L., Adams, A. L., and Klings, M., Fed. Proc.,
      Fed. Amer. Soc. Exp. Biol., 30, 1494 (1971).

22.   Booyse, F. M., and Rafelson, M. E., Jr., Ser. Haematol.,
      4, 152 (1971).

23.   Schoen, F., Fed. Proc., Fed. Amer. Soc. Exp. Biol., 30,
      1647 (1971).

24.   Baier, R. E. and Zobel, C. R., Nature, 212, 351 (1966).

25.   Loeb, G. I. and Baier, R. E., J. Colloid Interface Sci.,
      27, 38 (1968).

26.   Baier, R. E. and Loeb, G. I., in Polymer Characterization:
      Interdisciplinary Approaches, C. D. Craver, Ed., Plenum
      Press, New York, 1971.

27.   Kolobow, T., Stool, E. W., Weathersby, P. K., Pierce, J.,
      Hayano, F., and Suaudeau, J., Trans. Amer. Soc. Artif.
      Intern. Organs, 20, 269 (1974).

28.   Dahlquist, C. A., Hendricks, J. A., and Sohl, W. E.,
      U. S. Patent 2,532,011 (1950).

29.   Ward, C. A., Ruegsegger, B., Stanga, D., and Zingg, W.,
      Trans. Amer. Soc. Artif. Intern. Organs, 20, 77 (1974).

POROUS POLYMERIC ORTHOPEDIC IMPLANTS

Samuel F. Hulbert and L. S. Bowman

Tulane University, New Orleans, Louisiana, and
Medical University of South Carolina, Charleston,
South Carolina

The use of polymer sponges as non-weight-bearing bone
prostheses has received some degree of investigation. Encouraged
by reports on the successful use of polyvinyl sponge, a polymer
made by treating polyvinyl alcohol with formaldehyde and sulfuric
acid, Struthers [1] in 1955, tested its compatibility with soft tissue and bone. Using nine young adult dogs, he placed the material
in the periosteal bed of the ribs, the sternum, and in the rectus
abdominis muscle. He reported that bone ingrowth occurred within four weeks of implantation, and that the addition of chips or
small particles of autogenous bone to the implant increased the
extent of ingrowth. Histologic evaluation revealed that no foreign
body reaction had occurred up to a period of 20 weeks after implantation.

In 1958, Amler, et al. [2] carried out an experimental study
of polyvinyl sponge using adult albino rats. A trough, 5 mm long,
2 mm wide and 0.5 mm deep into the marrow cavity was prepared
in the dorsal aspect of the femur. It was found that when contact
between the sponge and the marrow cavity was established, a
structural attachment resulted and new bone infiltrated the sponge
in four weeks, increasing in amount up to 24 weeks. Moreover,
85% of the sponge had been resorbed after 12 weeks of implantation.

That same year, Bryan, et al. [3] reported the results of
polyvinyl sponge implants in 21 dog femora. They concluded that

161

this material, placed in cortical defects, definitely retards the process of bone healing, and can prevent complete healing for as long as one year.

In 1964, Barr, et al. [4] reported on osteogenic activity following implantation of polyvinyl sponge in 3 mm femoral defects of 30 mature guinea pigs. Initially, the implants deterred the formation of new tissue. These were compared with a control site in which no implant had been inserted. By ten days, osteoid was confirmed throughout the sponge, and by five weeks, all the defects were bridged. After eight weeks, the site of implantation was healed. The sponge was not completely removed, but was incorporated into the newly formed bone.

In 1958, Mandarino and Salvatore [5] reported the use of a polyurethane polymer which could be poured in liquid form and set up within 24 hours as a strong, nontoxic, cohesive aid in bone fracture repair. The polyurethane foam (ostamer) is prepared by reacting a trihydroxy resin with an excess of diisocyanate. This polymer is mixed with a catalyst at the time of surgery. Carbon dioxide is liberated, and a sponge-like compound of 7-10% cellular structure is produced. Defects were made in either the radius or femur of 66 dogs and filled with ostamer to bond the bone ends together. Complete bridging of the defect occurred in 80% of the cases.

After this promising experimental work, these same investigators [6] reported the use of ostamer in six clinical cases in 1959. The material was employed as a means of fixation in three nonunions, two pathologic fractures, and one acute fracture. The results over a three-year period were very successful, demonstrating that the material was well tolerated by the host, and that its strength of fixation was good. In 1960, Mandarino and Salvatore [7] reported the clinical use of ostamer in 220 cases, 93% of which were successful. They advocated its use in bone cysts, preamputation cases, and terminal malignancies with pathologic fractures.

Prompted by previous successful studies, Macoomb, et al. [8] evaluated the use of ostamer in experimental fractures of long bones in large animals, and the effect of this material on callus formation in healing fractures in rats. They found that ostamer did not act as a bone adhesive, as previous reports claimed, but rather as an intramedullary rod providing some measure of mechanical stability. The material evoked minimal tissue reaction.

There was, however, no histological evidence of osteoblastic activity within its framework.

The use of ostamer appeared to offer numerous advantages over conventional orthopedic methods, such as immediate and secure bone fixation, permitting rapid rehabilitation, and eventual replacement by host bone, eliminating the need for bone grafts. Predicated on these assumptions, Redler [9] employed this material in an experimental clinical study for treatment of a wide variety of orthopedic conditions in 42 patients. Fifty-one operations were performed on the 42 patients. There were nine successes, 37 failures, and five operations demonstrating clinically stable fixation but no radiographic evidence of bone union. Failure of fixation was attributed to the breaking of the polymer, or the loosening of the bond between polymer and bone. The operations were complicated by wound infection or by the development of a draining sinus in 21 of the 51 operations. The use of ostamer for osteosynthesis was therefore not recommended.

A more recent attempt to use plastic foams as bone substitutes was reported by McFall, et al. [10] in 1968. Acrylate amide foam (elastomer) was implanted supra- and subperiosteally in female albino rats. Elastomer is a polyacrylic ester rubber which is a terpolymer of 90 parts butyl acrylate, 7.5 parts methyl methacrylate, and 2.5 parts methacrylamide with 37 parts ethyl methacrylate filler. There was no evidence of significant alteration or resorption of elastomer during a 28-week period. Inflammation was present around and within the implanted sponge, but it subsided with time. It was concluded that the results justified further investigation in primates and human subjects.

Henefer, et al. [11] implanted elastomer in defects of the cancellous alveolar structures in 20 squirrel monkeys. The implants were tolerated up to 12 months, and no signs of active rejection occurred. New bone was formed in the spaces of the sponge and extended beyond the original contours of the labial cortical plate.

Polyethylene has a fairly long history as an implant material. Many of the early polyethylene implants consisted of the low density or low molecular weight material. These materials were, for the most part, used in plastic and reconstructive surgery to fill defects in both hard and soft tissue [12, 13, 14, 15, 16]. More recently, high density polyethylene (HDPE) and ultra-high molecular weight polyethylenes (UHMWPE) have been employed [17, 18, 19, 20, 21]. The widespread use of UHMWPE in orthopedic surgery originated with its utilization as an acetabular cup in hip arthroplasties. UHMWPE is currently being used in a wide variety of joint prostheses.

The ability of bone to grow into porous materials has been well demonstrated [22]. The concept of using this ingrown bone to anchor prostheses to the skeletal system is particularly appealing. Since polyethylene is presently used as a component of prosthetic joints and since a porous form of this material can be fabricated, a solid-porous polyethylene composite would seem to be well suited for joint reconstruction. The limited clinical studies conducted to date with porous polyethylene support the foregoing hypothesis [23].

Proplast, a porous polytetrafluoroethylene (Teflon) carbon fiber reinforced composite, has been successfully used clinically as a coating to allow for direct skeletal attachment via tissue ingrowth with temporomandibular condylar prostheses, femoral head prostheses, and endo-osseous blade-vent implants. In addition, Proplast as a bulk material has been placed subperiosteally to augment deficient mandibular alveolar ridge, shallow infraorbital and zygomatic prostheses, and deficient chins [24, 25].

Porous polyethylene and polytetrafluoroethylene appear to have bright futures as implant materials for direct skeletal stabilization via tissue ingrowth.

REFERENCES

1.   Struthers, A. M., Plast. Reconstr. Surg., 15, 274 (1955).

2.   Amler, M. H., Johnson, P. L., and Bevelander, G., Oral Surg., Oral Med., Oral Pathol., 11, 654 (1958).

3.   Bryan, R. S., Jones, J. M., and Grindlay, J. H., Proc. Mayo Clin., 33, 453 (1958).

4.   Barr, C. E., Salley, J. J., and LeHew, R. A., J. Dent. Res., 43, 26 (1964).

5. Mandarino, M. P. and Salvatore, J. E., Surg. Forum, 9, 762 (1958)

6. Mandarino, M. P. and Salvatore, J. E., Amer. J. Surg., 97, 442 (1959).

7. Mandarino, M. P. and Salvatore, J. E., Arch. Surg., 80, 623 (1960).

8. Macoomb, R. K., Hollenberg, C., and Zingg, W., Surg. Forum, 11, 454 (1960).

9. Redler, I., J. Bone Joint Surg., 44A, 1621 (1962).

10. McFall, T. A., Henefer, E. P., and Clinton, E. E., J. Oral Surg., 23, 108 (1965).

11. Henefer, E. P., McFall, T. A., and Hauschild, D. C., ibid., 26, 577 (1968).

12. Ingraham, F. D., Alexander, E. J., and Matson, D. P., J. Amer. Med. Assoc., 135, 82 (1947).

13. Brown, M. H., Grindlay, J. H., and Craig, W. K., Surg., Gynecol., Obstet., 86, 663 (1948).

14. Rubin, L. R., Robertson, G. W., and Shapiro, R. N., Plast. Reconstr. Surg., 3, 586 (1948).

15. Brush, E., Bing, J., and Hansen, E. H., Acta Chir. Scand. 97, 381 (1949).

16. Rubin, L. R., Plast. Reconstr. Surg., 7, 131 (1951).

17. Usher, F. and Gannon, J., Arch. Surg., 78, 131 (1959).

18. Usher, F. and Gannon, J., ibid., 78, 138 (1959).

19. Pennisi, V. R., Faggella, R. M., Ott, B. S., and Murphy, W. M., Plast. Reconstr. Surg., 30, 247 (1962).

20. Pennisi, V. R., Klabunde, E. H., McGregor, M., O'Connor, G. B., Pierce, G. W., and Faggella, R., ibid., 30, 254 (1962).

21.   Pennisi, V. R., Shapiro, R. L., Boucher, J. H., Pickens,
      G. E., and Shaddish, W. R., ibid., 35, 212 (1965).

22.   Klawitter, J. J. and Hulbert, S. F., J. Biomed. Mater.
      Res., 4, 571 (1970).

23.   Sauer, B. W., Weinstein, A. M., and Hopkins, J. E.,
      presented at the 6th International Biomaterials Symposium,
      Clemson, S. C., 1974.

24.   Hinds, E. C., Homsy, C. A., and Ken, J. N., presented at
      the 4th International Meeting of the Association of Oral
      Surgeons, Amsterdam, Holland, May, 1971.

25.   Kent, J. N., Homsy, C. A., Gross, B., and Hinds, E. C.,
      J. Oral Surg. 30, 608 (1972).

SKIN INTERFACING TECHNIQUES

C. Wm. Hall and J. J. Ghidoni

Southwest Research Institute, 8500 Culebra Road,
San Antonio, Texas 78284, and The University of Texas
Medical School at San Antonio, Pathology Department,
7703 Floyd Curl Drive, San Antonio, Texas 78229

The use of cables, lead wires and conduits to transmit signals and power from implanted devices to externally located devices requires penetration of and interfacing with the integument. Likewise the development of a bioadherent dressing for burn wound cover or development of a permanently placed artificial limb, requires interfacing of a foreign material with viable skin. In order to better understand the problem, a brief review of some of the important functions of the skin and its method of wound healing is in order.

The integument of our bodies which we call skin comprises the largest organ of the body both in surface area and in mass. Its most important function is simply a bag to contain all our body parts. As such, it also protects these parts from drying out and constitutes our first line of defense against microbial invasion. Both excretory and secretory glands are contained in this complex organ and these help regulate the body's fats, water and electrolytes. Evaporation of perspiration dissipates much of the body's heat and accounts for a large percentage of the insensible water loss. Our skin is our most extensive sense organ for the reception of thermal, tactile and painful stimuli.

When a break in the integument occurs, there is always some bleeding from the torn capillaries and oozing from intracellular interstitial fluids. A coagulum of cellular debris, fibrin and bacteria eventually forms which hardens to form an eschar. Beneath

167

the eschar an exciting series of events begin to take place. Poly-
morphoneuclear leukocytes first appear to clean house. These
plus the bacteria, nonviable tissue and foreign material are de-
lineated from the viable cells to become the base of the eschar.
At about the same time, fibrocytes invade the area and new vessels begin to form to become the granulating bed upon which new
epithelium will grow. Epithelial tissue has a tendency to cover
denuded areas by peripheral overgrowth. Only when the epithelial
cells meet and join with other epithelial cells, does this force
stop - its appetite for wandering finally satisfied. This is also
true of penetrating openings kept open by a rod or conduit - resulting in a sinus tract.

Finally, after the wound has been completely covered by epithelial cells, the granulating bed matures with some loss of capillaries and the fibrocytic portion of the granulating bed begins to
contract. Contraction of the resultant scar depends on many things,
among which are the size and shape of the original wound and the
required motion of the new skin.

Common injuries to the skin are puncture, lacerations, abra-
sions, evulsions and burns. Only the latter is of concern to us
here since burns often require prolonged and staged medical therapy for which a long-term bioadherent wound covering might be
applicable. As mentioned previously, other requirements for
epithelial interfacing in addition to a bioadherent dressing are to
allow penetrating rods, lead wires and conduits to remain in place
for prolonged periods of time without resulting in a sinus tract and
subsequent bacterial invasion. Such devices are needed for arteriovenous shunts used in long-term hemodialysis, as a linkage between an implanted artificial heart and an externally located power
supply and as a direct skeletal extension for a permanently attached
artificial limb. Discussion of the methods of selecting a suitable
material for these purposes and the appropriate fabricated configuration is the purpose of this paper.

When implanted within a biologic system, some materials are
relatively nonreactive, whereas others cause severe tissue responses. Hyperreaction in the form of fibrous hyperplasia is sometimes desirable, particularly if a firm bond between the tissue and
the foreign material is required. Such a bond is needed to satisfy
the requirements of the devices mentioned earlier. Therefore,
those materials which cause little or no tissue response should not
be considered for these purposes. Caution should be exercised in

formulating standards for implantable materials so as not to re-
strict those materials for usage where a certain type of tissue reaction is desirable. For this same reason, considerable thought
will be required in defining such terms as "biocompatible" and
"tissue compatibility" [1].

One of our early experiments was to test various polymers,
all of which were woven in a warp knit velour configuration. Polymers tested were Teflon, polypropylene, Dacron, nylon and rayon.
Each test fabric was backed with Silastic to form a laminate that
was to act as an "artificial skin" [2]. A 5x10 cm area of skin was
removed from the dorsum of a large number of canines, and replaced with one of the test laminates. Each laminate was held in
place with interrupted sutures tied over a stent dressing. In every
instance there was good tissue ingrowth into the interstices of the
velour, and as long as the sutures remained in place, the laminate
remained in position. However, once the sutures were removed,
the Teflon and polypropylene velours could easily be peeled off the
granulating bed. Considering the rate of attachment, rayon was
the earliest to adhere and the most tenacious. However, after ten
to 14 days the rayon velour disappeared, leaving only the Silastic
backing. For prolonged application, it too cannot be considered.
Dacron and nylon did not degrade and were held to the tissue with
about the same tenacity as rayon. Since all the velours tested had
the same geometric configuration, their mechanical attachments to
tissue were identical. The increase in bond strength must therefore be due to something other than the mechanical bond.

What is the common denominator which causes these two polymers to seemingly join hands with the surrounding tissue? Actually
we do not know the answer to this question, but we have postulated
that it is due to their hydrogen bonding ability and presumably they
share hydrogen atoms with the protein molecules.

The purpose of developing a bioadherent burn wound dressing
was to be able to hold a clean granulating bed in a state of readi-
ness until definitive autologous grafting could proceed. Although
this type of dressing has found application in immediate covering
of a burn wound, this was not its original purpose.

Clinical experience [3, 4, 5] has shown Dacron or nylon velour laminated with an appropriate material to (1) maintain a clean
granulating bed in a state of acceptance, (2) impede fluid and electrolyte losses from the wound and (3) almost completely abolish the

pain associated with this type of wound. Such wounds, when covered with a bioadherent dressing, require no further dressing
change until such time as a donor site becomes available for split
thickness autologous skin grafting.

A review of the literature along these lines will not be given
here. Interested readers are referred to previous papers by the
author [2, 3, 4, 5, 6] .

Interrupting the continuity of the integument in order to position rods, lead wires and conduits involves similar problems, and
consequently the same approaches as those encountered in developing a bioadherent dressing can be used.

The development of an exteriorized arteriovenous shunt
cannula suitable for hemodialysis has two diametrically opposed
requirements. The first is an inner surface which will interface
with blood so as to cause no tissue reaction (specifically, no
thrombosis), and a second requirement demands tissue reactivity
in order to obtain a firm bond with the integument. A nonreactive
outer surface on such a cannula is doomed to failure because of
the fact that ultimately a sinus tract will form which allows bacteria access to the cannulated vessels and subsequently results in
a phlebothrombosis.

Our concern was to develop a suitable outer surface which
would interface with the epithelium. * Any of the currently acceptable nonthrombogenic inner surfaces can be incorporated at a later
date. The experimental design actually used Silastic rods rather
than cannulae.

Various types of materials were bonded to the surface of these
Silastic rods and the rods implanted into the dorsum of canines,
goats and swine. At weekly intervals, the presence or absence of
the test rods was recorded and the condition of the wounds was
noted.

Materials bonded to the test rod and the results of these tests
appear in the table on the next page.

*Supported by National Institute of Arthritis and Metabolic
Diseases, Contract NIH-NIAMD-70-2109

Material	Results
1. Nylon velour Dacron velour	Excellent, only problem is eventually extrusion of rod - "Growth Phenomenon".
2. Polypeptide with rough cast surface or nonwoven fabric	Good for short-term usage but is biodegradable.
3. Polyurethane foam	Good for short-term usage but not as predictable as nylon velour.
4. Nylon foam	Poor. Probably due to closed cell construction of foam material.
5. Vitreous carbon buttons	No wound infections seen but excisional biopsies demonstrated complete marsupialization of implant.
6. Solid uncoated Silastic rod (used as control)	Sinus tract invariably formed. Could always be easily withdrawn when retaining suture was removed.

In general it was felt that foams were less predictable than the velour fabrics probably because of numerous dead spaces which were prone to become a nidus for infection. Carbon buttons cause no tissue reaction, give no bond to epithelial tissue, are always marsupialized and have no place as a potential skin interfacing material. This leaves velour and felt fabrics as the only potential materials to solve this problem.

It should be noted that porous ceramic has been advocated as a skin interfacing material by Hulbert, Klawitter and others. Although we have had no experience with porous ceramic other than as a bone interfacing material, we would anticipate some problems due to an impedence mismatch and dead spaces similar to foamed plastics.

As noted in the above summation, the velour fabrics have specialized problems of their own. Epithelium coming in contact with nylon or Dacron velour appears to satisy its desire to join with other epithelial tissue. A tenacious, mechanical-chemical bond between the basal epithelial layer and the velour is maintained as a permanent "marriage" during the maturation, migration and death of the individual epithelial cells. This results in a "growth phenomenon" causing the velour to migrate with the maturing epithelial cells. This is more noticeable on the dorsum of test animals than on the ventral surface or the limbs. Presumably this is due to a difference in the rate of maturation from one anatomical site to another. Our clinical experience has thus far involved shorter time intervals and perhaps explains our failure to duplicate this "growth phenomenon" in humans.

Our experience in developing a permanently attached artificial limb parallels in most respects the results outlined for the arteriovenous shunt cannulae. Here, of course, we must make an absolutely perfect bond with the skin in order to maintain a bacteria-proof seal. If this is not accomplished, osteomyelitis invariably results.

One thing is certain: epithelial tissue has an inborn desire to be joined on its free edge to other epithelial cells. Given the proper environment, it will continue to grow in hopes of a chance meeting with another epithelial edge to satisfy this dictum.

REFERENCES

1. Hall, C. W., J. Biomed. Mater. Res., Symp. No. 2, Pt. 1, 1 (1972).

2. Hall, C. W., Liotta, D., and DeBakey, M. E., Trans. Amer. Soc. Artif. Intern. Organs, 12, 340 (1966).

3. Hall, C. W., Spira, M., Gerow, F., Adams, L., Martin, E., and Hardy, S. B., ibid., 16, 12 (1970).

4. Spira, M., Hall, C. W., and Hardy, S. B., in Proceedings of the 3rd International Congress for Research in Burns, Prague, Czechoslovakia, 1970.

5.   Spira, M. and Hall, C. W., in Treatment of Burns,
     Proceedings of the Symposium of the Educational Foundation
     of the American Society of Plastic and Reconstructive Surgeons,
     Inc. with the cooperation of the American Burn Association,
     J. B. Lynch and S. R. Lewis, Eds., Vol. 5, 1973, p. 182.

6.   Hall, C. W., Liotta, D., Ghidoni, J. J., DeBakey, M. E.,
     and Dressler, D. P., J. Biomed. Mater. Res., 1, 179 (1967).

POLYMERS IN THE GENITOURINARY TRACT

Hans H. Zinsser

College of Physicians and Surgeons, Columbia
University, New York, N. Y.

In discussing biological compatibility of various natural and
synthetic materials on prolonged contact with the lining of the
genitourinary system, it is germane to discuss a little of what we
know of the secretions flowing through the genitourinary tract.

Urine itself represents a complex mixture of electrolytes, a
large quantity of urea, many organic acids, and bases to enumer-
ate some of the more than 170 small molecular weight components
[1]. Among the higher molecular weight materials, acid mucoproteins and neutral mucoproteins have been studied extensively
[2]. One intriguing mucoprotein, the Tam-Horsfall protein, is
precipitated by normal saline. It was originally thought to be secreted by the bladder trigone but has since been shown to come
from the upper tract [3]. In addition, the urine contains many
enzymes, among them β-glucuronidase, alkaline phosphatase, and
amylase.

The lower urinary tract in the male carries continuous weep-
ing or prostatic, seminal vesicular epididymal and testicular fluid
which includes quantities of citric acid, a potent fibrinolysin, a
potent lipase, and mucous secretions of the urethral lining. In the
female, only mucous from the urethral lining is added to the urinary load.

The urinary tract, particularly the distal 3 cm of the urethra,
is continuously the site of habitation of multiple viruses, pleuro-

175

pneumonia-like organisms, and bacteria. Many of these bacteria
can be found on the perineal skin and in the rectal area as well as
in the distal urethra. The most common invaders of the urinary
tract are the patient's own bacteria, usually passing down from
his own intestinal tract [4].

Bacteria in the urine may acidify the urine or alkalinize it.
Normal urine pH is between 5 and 6, but this may be made even
lower by some types of infection such as some of the salmonella.
More commonly, and more to be feared, are those organisms that
alkalinize the urine, chiefly through the mechanism of splitting
urea to two ammonia molecules and one carbon dioxide. After an
elevated urinary pH is attained, many insoluble precipitates form
in the urine; the commonest of these is a complex mixture of magnesium ammonium phosphate, calcium carbonate, and calcium
silicate.

Until the advent of organic material diuretics [5], we were
powerless to control this alkalinizing effect with oral or parenteral
medication.

The most disastrous interaction between the secretions of the
genitourinary tract occurs when they come into contact with polymers. This is a function of their urea content and urea splitting
propensity.

The lining of the urinary tract is far from an inactive membrane; it has complex secreting properties of its own. The first
experiments on anomalous osmosis were done with segments of
frog bladder [6]. The capacity of the bladder lining to resist re-
absorption of various urinary components is highly developed and
has been well studied. The bladder lining itself has been shown to
have phagocytic properties and much of its integrity is destroyed
by being overstretched.

Normal bladder tissue has not as yet been grown in tissue
culture and even low grade papillomas are difficult to maintain.
There is a strain of embryonic bladder cells which have been used
as a test system for the compatibility of various plastics with the
bladder lining. Whether these represent a true test system or not,
only further experience can tell. The earliest good results with
the growing of bladder tumor tissue were obtained in the anterior
chamber of the rabbit eye.

Study of the behavior of polymers that have been placed in contact with the urinary mucous membranes has taught us much about the disasters of allowing unreacted monomer to remain in contact with the lining. Many of these unreacted monomers are extremely reactive and lead to burns and scarification, and subsequent stricture formation in the urinary tract. In the early stages of development, polyvinyl chloride tubes for feeding infants were the worst offenders.

For a time, unreacted vulcanizing agents in rubber latex catheters were felt to be antibacterial, but shortly thereafter proved also to be violently irritative to the lining of the membrane.

A totally different picture is presented, however, by the intentional attempt to create an antibacterial surface on plastics using antibacterials shown to be compatible with mucous membranes [7].

The British have used extensively a material called Hibitane, chemically chlorohexidine, as an antiseptic irrigating material, and we in turn have used it to impregnate catheters for long-term installation. The material is highly insoluble in saline solution and in urine so that it tends to leach only very slowly out of the catheter.

In a series of 19 patients in which this antibacterial agent was used, excellent bacteriostasis was observed, but after the third instance of hematuria, we were forced to discontinue its use permanently.

Another material utilized with success has been Hexetidine, again a highly insoluble material, but more soluble in rubber latex than in urinary secretions. It was initially marketed as a mouthwash. It precipitates out onto the surface of the teeth and tongue, and leaves a long lasting antibacterial layer in its wake. This is formulated only in a mouthwash called Sterisol and, until recently, was available from the Lactona Division of Warner Lambert. Catheters soaked in this for 45 minutes and then washed in sterile saline prior to insertion have remained uninfected and uninvolved with deposits or concretions for over six to eight weeks in some patients. One patient who has been subjected to this type of prophylactic therapy has remained free of concretions for more than 15 years.

As intermittent catheterization becomes more widely applied, these necessities will be greatly reduced [8].

Polymers may be roughly sub-divided into two categories:

1. Easily wettable
2. More difficultly wettable, depending on the inter-
    facial tension between water and the plastic.

The most easily wettable are undoubtedly the hydrogels. These
are followed by some of the highly polymerized gelatins which have
been used for making tissue glues by reacting resorcinol, formaldehyde or more conveniently, homocystinethiolactone with the
gel. These gelatins are firm at body temperature and are completely biodegradable; they have not as yet been adequately investigated, but are of high potential utility. Rubber latex with or without ferric oxide filler has hydrophilic properties and is very rapidly wetted by water. Radioactive silver has been electrophoresed
into rubber latex [9]; studies of antibacterial properties have not
been made.

Those plastics which have been used in the urinary tract and
thought to be unwettable, such as polyethylene, polypropylene, silicone, Teflon, or polyurethane polyethers, are, in the presence of
lipoproteins, urea, mucoprapteins and bacteria, very promptly
coated with a wettable layer after their insertion into the urinary
tract. Concretions secondary to urea-splitting bacteria will not
adhere as firmly to silicone or Teflon, but their use is no guarantee
against the formation of surface concretions. In the experimental
laboratory, we have managed to produce magnesium ammonium
hydroxide precipitates on all plastics tested up to now, with the use
of urea-splitting bacteria. We have similarly been able to prevent
this with a variety of pretreatments, namely, either per os in the
rat, or by the type of treatment given to the plastic before insertion.

Slow degradation of silicone placed in the vas deferens was
shown to occur in experiments in the hog [10], and were in part
attributed to the fact that the polymerization may not have been
carried out adequately within the confines of the vas deferens.
Early work by Dr. Furey [11] in attempting to duplicate the results
of Dr. Murphy and coworkers [12] with the Holter valve in the ure-
ter showed that even in the absence of infection, the mechanical
properties of the silicone valve leaflets were significantly changed,
to the detriment of function, by the urea concentration alone. With
the recent publicity on the degradation of silicone cardiac valves in
the circulatory system, we are justified in exploring the possibility
that other plastics may be better than silicone when in body contact.

At present, it is planned to utilize polyurethane polyether plugs in the vas deferens. Animal experience is both extensive and encouraging [13].

REFERENCES

1. Stern, F., Grumet, G., Trabel, F., Mennis, A., and Zinsser, H. H., J. Chromatogr., 19, 130 (1965).

2. Gabriel, O., Dain, J., Zinsser, H. H., and Dische, Z., Arch. Biochem. Biophys., 86, 155 (1960).

3. Dische, Z., Kawasaki, H., Rothschild, C., Danilchenko, A., and Zinsser, H. H., ibid., 107, 209 (1964).

4. Kimmelman, L. J., Zinsser, H. H., and Klein, M., J. Urol., 65, 668 (1951).

5. Zinsser, H. H., Seneca, H., Light, I., Mayer, G., McGeoy, G., and Tarrasoly, H., N. Y. State J. Med., 68(6), 743 (1968).

6. Höber, R., Hitchcock, D. I., Bateman, J. B., Goddard, D. R., and Fenn, W. O., Physical Chemistry of Cells and Tissues, The Blakiston Company, Philadelphia, Pa., 1945.

7. Zinsser, H. H., Arouni, T. J., Schwartz, R., Trans. Amer. Soc. Artif. Intern. Organs, 5, 319 (1959).

8. Perkash, I., Intermittent Catheterization of the Paralyzed Bladder After Spinal Cord Injury, Urology Times, June, 1974, p. 3.

9. Zinsser, H. H., Wolf, J., Wertz, E., Uson, A., Goodwin, W., Al Waidh, M., and Azar, H., Radiology, 84, 428 (1965).

10. Hrdlicka, G., and Zinsser, H. H., Fertil. Steril., 18, 289 (1967).

11. Furey, C., J. Urol., 85(4), 525 (1961).

12. Murphy, J. J., Rattner, W. H., and Schoenberg, H., ibid.,
    <u>82</u>, 481 (1959).

13. Boretos, J. W. and Pierce, W. S., J. Biomed. Mater. Res.,
    <u>2</u>, 121 (1968).

BIOLOGICAL MODEL SYSTEMS FOR THE TESTING OF THE TOXICITY OF BIOMATERIALS

John Autian

Materials Science Toxicology Laboratories, College of Pharmacy and College of Dentistry, The University of Tennessee, Center for the Health Sciences, Memphis, Tennessee 38163

INTRODUCTION

An increasing number of medical items, classified as medical devices, are being manufactured, distributed and used for the saving of lives, prolongation of life, and in all aspects of health care. These items can range from heart valves to disposable plastic syringes. Presently, it is estimated that approximately 3,000 to 4,000 firms are manufacturing approximately 20,000 medical devices of one type or another. The 1974 market value for these items is estimated to range from $3 billion to $5 billion, and this figure is expected to increase significantly in the next five years.

Even though a medical device law still has not been passed by Congress, there appears to be no doubt that within a short period of time an acceptable medical device act will become a reality, and much more rigid controls will be imposed upon the medical device industry in regard to efficacy and safety of its particular line of items.

Since many medical items are composed partly or completely of man-made polymeric materials, metal alloys and in some cases ceramics, and since, in many cases, these items will have either direct or indirect contact with patients, all possible steps should be taken to ensure that these items do not release a chemical entity to the patient which can lead to undesirable effects. The proper use of selected toxicity or safety tests with appropriate biological models can lead to the rejection of potentially harmful materials while permitting the safe materials to be considered for the manufacture of a medical device.

One must also recognize that the specific end use of the device will also play a part in the types and numbers of biological tests which a manufacturer should perform to establish the safety of his item. Table I illustrates an oversimplified classification of medical items, based upon end use. From what has already been said, it is clear that there will be a need for the manufacturer to conduct toxicity tests and studies at the materials level (selection of a specific material for the specific device), and on the final device. It should be appreciated that, for a new material and a new device, the tests and studies will generally be more extensive and more time-consuming than those which will eventually be used as quality control procedures once the product has been placed on the market.

The principal purpose of this presentation is to discuss the most suitable preclinical testing procedures for all biomaterials to help indicate if leachable biologically active constituents are actually released. Brief comments will first be made on classical approaches in use today for the evaluation of safety or toxicity of chemical agents. The reader should understand that the art and science of toxicology for the evaluation of chemical agents (and various types of physical forces) are fairly extensive and growing rapidly, and those desiring more extensive review of this subject should turn to books or other publications on toxicity.

SOME GENERAL CONSIDERATIONS IN THE TESTING OF CHEMICALS

Preclinical Testing

For specific chemical agents, toxicological testing or safety testing programs are divided classically into three categories: (1) acute toxicity, (2) subacute toxicity, and (3) chronic toxicity. Each of these categories will be touched upon briefly in the sections to follow.

TABLE I

CLASSES OF PLASTIC DEVICES ACCORDING TO USE*

Class	Device or Item	Examples
1	Permanent implants	Heart valves, various vascular grafts, orthopedic implants, other artificial organs, etc.
2	Implants having contact with mucosal tissue	Artificial eyes, contact lens, dentures, intrauterine devices, certain types of catheters.
3	Corrective, protective, and supportive devices	Splinters, braces, films, protective clothes, etc.
4	Collection and administration devices	Blood transfusion sets, various types of catheters, dialyzing units, hypodermic devices and similar injection devices, etc.
5	Storage devices	Containers, bags for blood, blood products, drug products, nutritional products, diagnostic agents, etc.

*Reproduced from Autian, J., J. Dent. Res., 45, 1668 (1966).

Acute toxicity. One of the most important concepts in acute
toxicity is the dose-response relationship. In other words, the
term implies that at different dose levels, different intensities of
response can be observed. For practically all cases, as the dose
is increased, the intensity of the biological event being measured
will also increase, leading to a maximum effect which may be
death of the experimental animals. In any acute toxicity testing
program, it is assumed that the animals have been exposed to the
chemical only once. Depending upon the intended use of the chemical, a series of test procedures may be employed to establish the
harmful effect of the chemical as related to a dose or concentration
of the agent administered to the animals. The tests generally will
include experiments which will discern the lethality of the chemical when administered by several routes such as oral, dermal or
actual injection into the body. In most instances the toxicologist
will take his lethality data and, by a simple statistical procedure,
calculate the LD_{50} (the dose or concentration which will kill 50%
of the animals in the experiment).

A number of well-established test procedures are available
for determining the acute toxicity of chemicals. These can range
from the irritant effect of a chemical on the skin to behavioral
changes brought about by the chemical when administered to test
animals. In more recent years, sensitization tests have also been
included with acute toxicity tests, even though in some quarters
this type of test is generally included under the broad category of
subacute toxicity.

Subacute toxicity. For many chemical agents, however, it is
also necessary to know the toxic effects when animals are exposed
repeatedly to the specific chemical. Again as for acute toxicity
studies, similar biological responses can be measured and related to a specific dose or concentration administered to the test
animals. Generally, studies falling into this subacute toxicity
category will last from several weeks up to approximately three
months. A well-designed subacute toxicity study will include a
rather large number of test procedures which will reveal the dose
level at which the first toxic signs or symptoms occur. If these
studies are conducted in several species of animals, the toxicologist can generally rationalize a "no effect" dose or, stating this
another way, that dose which can be considered safe to humans
when these individuals have continual or repeated exposure to the
chemical lasting up to three months.

Chronic toxicity. Chronic toxicity studies imply that a chemical agent will be investigated in animals over a long period of time
where the animals receive repeated doses of the compound by one
or more routes of administration. Essentially, the tests used for
subacute toxicity are employed for the chronic toxicity studies and
again a "no effect" dose is determined.

Special tests and studies. For many chemical agents, it is
now necessary to include additional tests or studies which even a
decade ago were generally not conducted. These include studies
which will reveal the carcinogenic, teratogenic, and mutagenic
effects of the agents. In many cases, these types of studies will
depend upon the specific end use of the chemical, and thus, may
be incorporated into subacute or chronic toxicity studies.

At times the toxicologist may find that one or more in vitro
test may be useful in the study of the toxicity of a new chemical.
For example, various types of tissue culture procedures are receiving more attention as toxicity tools to study the effect of the
test compound at the cellular level. Isolated organs (such as the
heart, intestine, lungs, etc.) used to detect the effect of the chemical on these body systems can also be employed where end use
conditions suggest the information to be pertinent.

Clinical Studies

Predictions can be made from the various preclinical testing
programs as to the expected toxic effect of a chemical in humans
and the dose levels where the toxic effects are essentially manifested. Since one cannot be certain what effects a chemical will
have upon man, it may be necessary to examine the effects of the
agent in a direct manner such as by administration of the compound to selected groups of persons under close supervision of a
medical team. Clinical information on the toxicity of chemicals
can also come through epidemiological studies or through the examination of individual and collective health records. Included
may be those which industrial groups maintain on their employees
and information from various hospitals treating patients who have
been exposed, either accidentally or intentionally, to an agent
producing intoxication or death.

SOME GENERAL CONSIDERATIONS ON THE
TOXICITY TESTING OF BIOMATERIALS

The testing of chemical agents for the evaluation of the toxicity or safety of the agent is briefly presented in the foregoing discussion. Tests range from those used for the evaluation of acute toxicity to those which help to reveal the chronic toxicity of the agent under specified experimental procedures. It is also pointed out that clinical testing for toxicity may be required for certain chemicals, and that additional clinical toxicity information may be obtained from health records of workers exposed to specific chemicals, or from hospital records of patients having been intoxicated by a chemical agent.

A toxicologist entering the field of materials toxicology must utilize and develop new testing procedures or adapt the more classical toxicity testing procedures to the evaluation of safety or toxicity of a new biomaterial. If the biomaterial is to come into contact with the skin or mucous membranes, or be implanted into the body, answers to the following questions must be obtained:

1. Will the material produce an irritant response at the site of contact with tissue?

2. Will the material, through the release of a chemical constituent, produce a systemic toxic reaction?

3. Will the material act as an allergenic agent?

4. Will the material interact with cellular constituents to bring about an untoward effect?

5. Will the material remain stable in the body environment for the period of intended contact or implantation?

Unfortunately, the toxicologist cannot readily dissolve these materials in a suitable vehicle in order to appraise the dose-response relationship as can be done for chemical agents. He must be content to use the material as such, or to prepare extracts which in turn can be studied in biological systems.

A number of medical devices may not actually come in contact with tissue directly, but because drugs and various types of fluids (such as blood and blood products) may be stored, collected or administered in these devices, it is possible that extractable constituents from the biomaterials of the device will be administered to patients. The first three questions raised for biomaterials in contact with tissue are still valid for devices which may release chemical constituents to the solutions in contact with them.

Sound and comprehensive toxicity testing programs for medical devices should most likely be carried out at three levels of investigation:

Level I : A series of preclinical tests and studies in animals and in vitro systems.

Level II : An "in-use" test(s) in animals which would attempt to simulate the human use of the medical device.

Level III: Clinical trials in humans.

Only Level I testing will be discussed here. This initial phase of testing would be applicable to the final material to be used in the medical device. Level II and III testing procedures need to be developed for groups of devices having similar applications. Up to the present time, well-developed testing protocols for these two levels of testing are not available; therefore, each manufacturer must formulate his own protocol.

LEVEL I TESTING PROGRAM

In the Materials Science Toxicology (MST) Laboratories, a number of toxicity test procedures have been developed and used along with existing test procedures, both of which can be included in Level I testing. These test procedures are listed in Table II. As will be noted, the tests are divided into four general categories. They include (1) acute toxicity or screening tests, (2) subacute toxicity tests, (3) chronic and carcinogenic tests, and (4) special tests. At the present time it is felt that each of the tests listed under acute toxicity (Table II) should be employed for a completely new biomaterial and that selected tests from the same group can

TABLE II

LEVEL I TOXICITY TESTING OF BIOMATERIALS

A. Acute Toxicity or Screening Tests
    1. Tests Directly on Material
        a. Tissue culture - agar overlay method
        b. Rabbit muscle implant, USP
        c. Hemolysis (rabbit blood)

    2. Tests on Saline and Cottonseed Oil Extracts
        a. Tissue culture - agar overlay method
        b. Tissue culture - cell growth inhibition
            (distilled water used as extracting
            medium)
        c. Hemolysis (rabbit blood)
        d. Intracutaneous injection in rabbits, USP
        e. Systemic toxicity in mice, USP

B. Subacute Toxicity Tests
    1. Twelve-Week Rabbit Implantation

    2. Guinea Pig Maximization Test (for sensitization)

    3. Thirty-Day Systemic Toxicity Test

C. Chronic Toxicity and Carcinogenic Tests

D. Special Tests

then be employed when quality control procedures are developed.
It is of course understood that if the medical device is to be sterile
and nonpyrogenic, appropriate tests (not included here) must also
be employed.

Subacute toxicity tests should be considered for those biomaterials which will have short-term contact with tissue, while chronic
toxicity and carcinogenic studies will be necessary for those biomaterials which will have long-term contact, in particular, as implants.

In the category of special tests, it may be desirable to utilize
isolated rabbit heart experiments for those medical devices which
are destined for contact with drug products or various types of
alimentation fluids, or for medical items such as heart-lung machines and dialysis units.

The sections to follow will review the test procedures listed
in Table II. Published test methods are referenced. Some general comments for a number of the tests are made, and where
possible, the advantages and disadvantages are pointed out.

Acute Toxicity or Screening Tests

Tests directly on material. The tissue culture - agar overlay
assay is based on that described by Guess, et al. [1] and is designed to detect the response of a mammalian monolayer cell culture to readily diffusible components of materials or test solutions
applied to the surface of an agar layer overlaying the monolayer.

A 24-hour confluent monolayer is propagated in the bottom of
a Petri dish, and the liquid medium is aspirated and replaced by
a standard layer of agar containing the minimum nutrient requirements of the cells. The monolayer is stained with a vital dye,
neutral red, by application of a standard quantity of dye to the surface of the agar and aspiration of the excess from the agar surface
after a standard period of time.

Solid test samples, approximately 1 sq cm, are placed on the
surface of the agar. Each Petri dish receives two test samples
plus one positive control (known toxic material) and one negative
control (known nontoxic material). Powders (100 mg) are applied

directly to the agar surface covering an area of approximately
1 sq cm. After application of the test samples, the Petri dishes
are placed in a 37°C incubator for 24 hours (5% carbon dioxide
atmosphere).

The response of the cell monolayer is evaluated with respect
to the extent of decolorization of the red-stained monolayer under
and around the sample when the Petri dish is viewed against a
white background. Loss of color of the stained cells is considered
to be a physiologically significant reaction of the cells. The extent of decolorization is confirmed by examination of the monolayer on an inverted microscope and the extent of lysis of the cells
within the decolorized zone is estimated. Typically, decolorization of cells precedes lysis as manifested by a region of decolorized cells between a normal, fully stained region and a region
showing lysis. A sample is reported as cytotoxic only if lysis is
observed. The magnitude of the response of the monolayer may
be reported in terms of a Response Index:

RESPONSE INDEX = ZONE INDEX/LYSIS INDEX*

where the Zone Index is related to the size of the decolorized zone
and the Lysis Index is related to the extent of lysis within the zone
as defined below:

Zone index	Description of zone
0	No detectable zone around or under sample
1	Zone limited to area under sample
2	Zone not greater than 0.5 cm in extension from sample
3	Zone not greater than 1.0 cm in extension from sample
4	Zone greater than 1 cm in extension from sample, but not involving the entire plate
5	Zone involving the entire plate

---

*Ratio should not be reduced. The numerator and denominator
should remain as is.

Lysis index	Description of extent of lysis (microscopic)
0	No observable lysis
1	Less than 20% of the zone lysed
2	Less than 40% of the zone lysed
3	Less than 60% of the zone lysed
4	Less than 80% of the zone lysed
5	Greater than 80% lysed within the zone

This test method has been found to be an extremely useful and sensitive procedure to detect diffusible biologically active constituents from polymeric materials. It correlates highly with the USP rabbit implant procedure [2] but is more sensitive; thus, it is possible to report a negative response in the rabbit muscle while recording a cytotoxic response in the cell culture method. In all instances when a negative or toxic response is recorded in the rabbit implant, a cytotoxic response will be seen in the tissue culture procedure. In most instances it is adequate to report the tissue culture response as noncytotoxic or cytotoxic, but in other instances it may be beneficial to use the Response Index. This method of recording permits a greater sensitivity to be woven into this procedure. An increase in the numerical values in both numerator and denominator indicates an increase in the cytotoxic character of the material.

Should greater sensitivity be desired, the test samples can be placed directly on the cells (no agar), but this may add some disadvantages since certain materials can float on the surface, and thus move during the time required for incubation.

The rabbit muscle implant method appears in The United States Pharmacopeia [2] and may be considered as one of the simplest biological tests for detecting the leachable characteristics of a polymeric material.

Briefly, the test material is cut or formed into thin cylinders or rectangles measuring approximately 1.5 cm x 1 mm and is placed into the beveled point of a 15 G trocar needle having a length of 1.5 in. The needle is introduced into the paravertebral muscle and is then withdrawn, leaving the material implanted in the muscle. Two animals are used for each test material. A positive control (known toxic plastic) and a negative control (a known nontoxic material) are also implanted into the animals. After one week, the animals are sacrificed and the sites of the implants compared with the positive and negative controls. The macroscopic examination of the implant sites is then scored from 0 (nonreactive) to 3 (marked reaction). A questionable response is scored as $\pm$.

When necessary to confirm a toxic or irritant response, histopathology can be performed on the excised tissue surrounding the implant.

In the MST Laboratories, twelve histological criteria are examined for tissue response [3]. They include:

1.	Necrosis	7.	Giant cells
2.	Inflammation	8.	Foreign body debris
3.	Polymorphonuclear leukocytes	9.	Fibroplasia
4.	Macrophages	10.	Fibrosis
5.	Lymphocytes	11.	Fatty infiltration
6.	Plasma cells	12.	Relative size of involved area

Each of these criteria is then scored as follows:

0 = item not present
1 = item occasionally present
2 = item present to a mild degree
3 = item present to a marked degree

From these twelve items an overall toxicity rating of the test sample is assigned as follows:

0 = nontoxic
1 = very slight toxic reaction
2 = mild toxic reaction
3 = moderate toxic reaction
4 = marked toxic reaction

In the USP procedure, a positive control (or toxic test sample) is not necessary. The method used by the MST Laboratories includes a positive control which is plasticized polyvinyl chloride with 3.0% of an organotin compound used as a stabilizer.

For routine testing of biomaterials, the USP method without histopathology is quite adequate. This method, however, does not have the sensitivity of the tissue culture test described earlier, but sensitivity can be increased by the use of histopathology.

The MST Laboratories have found that, for acute toxicity, the residence time of implant should be seven days rather than three days as used by some laboratories. A three-day implant may reflect the physical trauma due to the insertion of the needle rather than the toxic effects of a leachable constituent from the material.

The hemolysis method utilizes fresh, whole oxalated rabbit blood, diluted sufficiently (usually 8 ml blood + 10 ml normal saline) so that when 0.2 ml is hemolyzed in 10 ml of 0.1% sodium carbonate solution, the spectrophotometric reading at 545 mμ will be about 10-13% transmission (1.0-0.9 optical density). For most materials, 5 g* cut, if necessary, into small pieces are placed in a 16 x 150 mm test tube, covered with 10 ml of normal saline, and placed in a 37°C water bath for 30 minutes to provide temperature equilibration. Then 0.2 ml of the diluted rabbit blood is added to the tube, mixed gently, and incubated for 60 minutes. The positive control is obtained by adding 0.2 ml of the diluted blood to 10 ml of 0.1% sodium carbonate solution, and the negative control is 0.2 ml of the diluted blood in 10 ml of normal saline (incubation time and other procedures are the same as for the test sample). After 60 minutes of incubation, all tubes are centrifuged for ten minutes at 500 x g, and the supernatant is carefully removed to prevent disturbing the precipitate, and then transferred to spectrophotometric cells.

Absorbance of each supernatant is determined at 545 mμ and recorded. The percent hemolysis is calculated as follows:

$$\% \text{ Hemolysis} = \left[\frac{(\text{O.D. test sample}) - (\text{O.D. negative control})}{(\text{O.D. positive control}) - (\text{O.D. negative control})} \right] \times 100$$

The percent hemolysis should be based upon the average of three replicates. If the hemolysis value is 5% or less, the material can be considered as being nonhemolytic under the experimental conditions employed.

---

*For certain types of materials such as fibers and threads it may be necessary to reduce the sample weight from 5.0 g to 0.5 g.

Tests on saline and cottonseed oil extracts. Test samples
are extracted following the procedure given in the USP [2]. Saline
solution and cottonseed oil are used as the extracting media. The
extraction is conducted at 121°C for one hour and the resultant extracts are set aside for biological testing. Tests on extracts
should be performed within 24 hours of completing the extraction
procedure. For the tissue culture - cell inhibition test, distilled
water is used as the extracting medium.

The tissue culture - agar overlay procedure is the same as
that described previously for solid test samples, except that 0.2 ml
of the extract is deposited on the surface of sterile paper discs
which have been previously placed on the agar. Two plates are
used for each extract and for each plate two paper discs with the
extract are included. A negative control (solvent alone) is also
included on each plate, as well as a positive control (toxic plastic
as in previous tissue culture method). The remainder of the procedure is exactly as that included in the previous section for tissue
culture.

For the tissue culture - cell growth inhibition test, only the
distilled water extract is used. Mouse fibroblast cells (strain
L-929) are monolayered in 32 oz culture bottles. The medium is
removed, the monolayer is trypsinized, and the cells are suspended in Eagle's medium. Cell density in the suspension is then
determined by hemocytometer count and is adjusted with Eagle's
medium to provide 1×10^5 cells/ml. Equal quantities of double
strength Eagle's medium and extract are mixed in sufficient quantity to permit the addition of 2 ml to each test tube in the extract-
treated series. Similarly, Eagle's medium and the extracting
medium (distilled water) are mixed for addition to the control tubes.
Two ml of standardized cell suspension is delivered to each of ten
test tubes (16 x 150 mm with stainless steel culture tube closures)
for the controls, and to ten test tubes to be used for the test samples (extract). All tubes containing the 2 ml of standardized cell
suspensions are then centrifuged aseptically and the medium aspirated from the packed cells. Two ml of Eagle's medium is added
to the ten control test tubes, and 2 ml of extract-treated medium
to each of the remaining ten tubes. At this point, the cells are resuspended by brief agitation on a vortex mixer. Five control tubes
and five extract-treated tubes are placed in the incubator for 72
hours. The remaining five controls and five extract-treated tubes
are centrifuged at 200 x g for five minutes and carefully decanted

in a manner to prevent loss of cells. The cells in the tubes are
carefully resuspended in 5 ml of normal saline, centrifuged, decanted taking care not to lose cells, and these tubes are then
stored at 4°C. These last sets of tubes serve to provide "zero"
time protein levels in subsequent calculation of cell growth.

After incubating for 72 hours, both controls and treated tubes
are centrifuged, and the medium is removed and washed with saline as described previously. The total protein content of each
tube is determined according to the procedure of Oyama and Eagle
[4] using the colorimetric method of Lowry, et al.[5] for protein
quantitation. The optical density (O.D.) is determined for each
tube (at 650 mμ) and an average O.D. is obtained for each set of
five tubes. Percent of inhibition of cell growth (%ICG) is then
calculated as shown:

$$\%ICG = 100 - 100 \times \frac{(O.D.\ 72\text{-hr treated tubes}) - (O.D.\ \text{zero time treated tubes})}{(O.D.\ 72\text{-hr control tubes}) - (O.D.\ \text{zero time control tubes})}$$

Since there is a linear relationship between cell number and
protein concentration, the percent inhibition of cell growth can be
calculated as shown from the formula. This method permits a
quantitative expression of the cytotoxicity of an extract (from a
biomaterial). Generally, extracts producing 5% ICG or less are
considered as being noncytotoxic extracts. The procedure described is perhaps the most sensitive method in the series of tests
listed in Table II under acute toxicity or screening tests. One
disadvantage of this test procedure is that it cannot be used for
nonaqueous systems and generally requires technical skill and
care to obtain accurate data.

To perform the hemolysis test, 10 ml of the saline extract is
placed in a test tube which in turn is inserted into a 37°C water
bath. After 30 minutes, 0.2 ml of diluted rabbit blood as described
in the previous section on hemolysis is added to the tube, and the
tube gently mixed and returned to the water bath for an additional
60 minutes. The tube is centrifuged and the supernatant removed
for the determination of percent hemolysis (method of calculation
given in previous section on hemolysis). This test is run in trip-
licate and the results averaged.

As with the previous hemolysis test on the material directly,
a hemolysis value of 5% or less is considered as being nonhemolytic.

The intracutaneous method is essentially that as described in the USP [2] with some minor modifications. Briefly, 0.2 ml of the extract is injected intracutaneously at ten sites on the dorsal surface of each of two rabbits, previously clipped of hair. The extract is injected on one side of the animal. On the other side, 20% ethyl alcohol is injected (0.2 ml) at five sites as a positive control, while five additional sites are injected (0.2 ml) with the extracting media. At 24, 48, and 72 hours the sites of injection for the extract are scored as compared to the controls. The scoring system ranges from 0 (similar to the negative control) to 3 (equal to the positive control).

This test procedure can reveal the irritant response of the extract. The sensitivity of this test is much less than that of tissue culture, but at times the cottonseed oil extract will demonstrate a rather marked irritant response. If information on the immediate irritant local response is desired, a vital dye may be used. For example, by injecting trypan blue intravenously fifteen minutes after the last test injection, irritant responses may be noted within the first hour. These immediate responses can be scored as compared to the controls. Extracts producing no greater irritancy than the negative control can be considered as passing this test.

The systemic toxicity method follows the USP procedure [2]; five mice are injected i.v. (saline) or i.p. (cottonseed oil or polyethylene glycol-400) at a dose level of 50 ml/kg. Five mice are injected with the extracting medium. All animals are observed at various time periods up to 72 hours. Signs of toxicity as well as deaths are recorded.

If the animals receiving the extract show no greater response than the control animals, the biomaterial can be considered not to have released toxic agents. In general, this procedure is not a very sensitive test and toxic results will be obtained only if the material has a very toxic substance which can diffuse into the extracting media. Any material producing a severe systemic toxic response (death) most likely should not be employed for a biomedical application.

Subacute Toxicity Tests

Twelve-week rabbit implantation. This method has been described in a publication by Turner, et al. [6]. The procedure follows that described for the USP rabbit implant. In the present test, however, 12 rabbits are implanted and one rabbit is sacrificed each week. The tissues of the implant sites are then excised and prepared for histopathologic examination. The results are recorded as given under the rabbit implant test described in a previous section.

For biomaterials which will have contact with tissue for short to moderate periods of time, this 12-week test appears appropriate since it documents a time-response profile which can be very helpful in judging the merits of a new biomaterial. When desired, this procedure can be extended to 6 or 12 months.

Guinea pig maximization test for sensitization. This procedure is an adaptation of that suggested by Magnusson and Kligman [7]. A detailed description of this test is presented.

Albino guinea pigs, preferably of the Hartley strain, weighing 300-500 g should be the test animals. A minimum of five guinea pigs should be used for each test compound. The authors, however, indicate that 25 guinea pigs would be more appropriate.

The guinea pig is lightly anesthetized with sodium pentobarbital (20 mg/kg). The anterior dorsal region of the thorax is shaved of hair and cleansed with 70% ethyl alcohol. In each animal, six intradermal injections are made, as pairs, 1-2 cm apart as illustrated:

```
         ┌─────────────────┐
         │ 1            1   │ . . . 0.1 ml Freund's adjuvant
         │                  │         without extract
Injection│ 2            2   │ . . . 0.1 ml of extract without
  region │                  │         Freund's adjuvant
         │ 3            3   │ . . . 0.1 ml of extract emulsified
         └─────────────────┘         in Freund's adjuvant
```

Injections using the adjuvant should be made slightly deeper to minimize sloughing of tissue. All animals are returned to their cages and observed daily for seven days.

One week after the initial injections (first stage), the second stage of induction is begun. The dorsal area used in the first stage is shaved again. If the extract is nonirritating, the region should be treated with 10% sodium lauryl sulfate in petrolatum to help provoke a mild inflammatory response. Twenty-four hours later, the extract is applied to a 2 x 4 cm patch of Webril cotton or a disc of filter paper, placed over the injection sites, and attached with an impermeable 3M Blenderm surgical tape (Minnesota Mining & Manufacturing Co., St. Paul, Minnesota). This patch is secured with an elastic bandage. After 48 hours, the dressing is removed and the area cleansed with 70% ethyl alcohol.

The challenging procedure is initiated two weeks following initiation of the second stage of induction. An unused site on the hind flank of the animal is chosen, shaved of hair, and cleansed with 70% ethyl alcohol. A patch containing the extract is applied to this area and bandaged as for the second stage of induction. Twenty-four hours later, the bandage and patch are removed. After an additional 24 hours, the area is cleansed with 70% ethyl alcohol and evaluated for an allergic reaction. The following scoring system is used:

> 0 = no reaction
> 1 = scattered mild redness
> 2 = moderate and diffuse redness
> 3 = intense redness and swelling

Based upon the number of animals sensitized, a rating of sensitization can be given as shown below:

Maximization Grading

% Sensitized	Grade	Classification
0 - 8	I	Weak
9 - 28	II	Mild
29 - 64	III	Moderate
65 - 80	IV	Strong
81 - 100	V	Extreme

This test procedure is more sensitive than the classical Draize test [8] for sensitivity. All new biomaterials should be screened through this type of test.

Thirty-day systemic toxicity test. Groups of 15 rats (male) are given the extract intraperitoneally at a dose of 25 ml/kg each day for 30 days. The extracting medium alone is administered to a control group of rats. During the test period, all animals are observed for weight gain/loss, general health, and mortalities. At the end of the 30 days, animals are sacrificed and the gross pathology is conducted on internal tissue and organs. Futher observations are made on selected tissues and organs by histopathologic examination.

Depending upon the final use of the biomaterial, this test can be expanded during the 30-day period to include other tests such as blood chemistry, urinalysis, hematology and organ function tests.

Chronic Toxicity and Carcinogenic Tests

The test material should be powdered or reduced to a particle size of less than 0.5 cm. The material (250 mg) is then implanted subdermally into the nape of 30 male black Bethesda rats, two to three months old. A similar group of rats is sham-operated and these serve as controls. All animals should be observed over a two-year period for deaths, toxic signs, and the development of tumors at implant sites or in remote areas.

Implants of powders or particles of less than 0.5 cm are used to reduce the incidence of solid-state tumors. If the test group of rats shows a significantly greater incidence of tumors at implant sites or in other areas, the material may be considered as a potential carcinogenic agent. This type of test should be considered for all new biomaterials which are anticipated to be left in the body for long periods of time ranging from several years to one or two decades.

Special Tests

Depending upon the end use of the biomaterial, there may be a need to utilize other test procedures not included in this discussion. One such test presently being used by the MST Laboratories

is based on an isolated rabbit heart response. Details of this test
will not be given here. The test, however, includes an extraction
procedure using Chenoweth's solution which can be circulated
through a device such as an artificial kidney for periods of time,
and then this solution is perfused into the isolated heart of a rabbit.
Effect on heart rate, amplitude, and coronary flow can be recorded
and the data compared to that of a Chenoweth's solution having no
contact with the device being tested. The isolated rabbit heart
test is an extremely sensitive test and is perhaps second only to
the tissue culture - cell growth inhibition test.

COMMENTS ON LEVEL I TESTING PROGRAM

With the use of a large battery of biological models as described here, questions may be raised as to which tests will be
the most relevant to clinical situations. Presently, there is no
conclusive answer and the judgment as to acceptance or rejection
of a new biomaterial must be based upon the final end use of the
device and the opinions of those who are testing the material. The
biological models used in the acute toxicity or screening tests
should be looked upon as those which help reveal if the test material has a diffusible chemical(s) which may have the propensity to
be harmful to patients. A broad range of biological models, rather
than one or two model systems, will permit greater confidence in
assessing a new biomaterial. For example, if the test material
did not produce toxic effects in any of the tests conducted, the conclusion could be reached that this specific material, when used
clinically, would probably not produce a harmful effect. On the
other hand, if the test material is found toxic by all tests employed,
then the conclusion would be that this material probably should not
be used for most biomedical devices.

Since the tests described in this presentation have various sen-
sitivities for the detection of biological responses, some materials
may be deemed "nontoxic" by one test system and "toxic" by another. In fact, it has already been indicated that the tissue culture
tests and the isolated heart experiments are much more sensitive
than other tests such as the rabbit implant, systemic toxicity, and
intracutaneous tests. How should the results of such tests be used
in making a judgment as to the acceptance or rejection of the test
material? In these situations a careful review should be made by
the investigator or manufacturer as to the final end use of the
medical device. If the material will not have contact with any

tissue, drug products, or various biological fluids, the more sensitive tests may in fact not be relevant, and a decision to reject an otherwise very good material may be premature. Final decisions for rejecting this "good" material should be based upon the assessment of the benefit-to-risk ratio for the final medical device. For example, if the device is a lifesaving one and no real substitute is available, the benefits to the patients can be far greater than any potential toxic effects found in a biological testing program. On the other hand, if several of the same type of lifesaving devices are available, the one not eliciting a toxic response should be the item employed.

Several of the biological tests falling in the area of the acute toxicity or screening tests appear appropriate for use in quality control procedures. In particular, the tissue culture tests can, when used properly, alert the manufacturer that contamination may have occurred in his biomaterial, and thus, the material should not be released until the causative agent is found and eliminated.

Even though it is generally desirable to utilize chemical and physical tests for the evaluation of the safety of a biomaterial or device, some reservations are in order. Experiences from the MST Laboratories have shown repeatedly that one cannot rely soley on a chemical analysis of extracts as the criterion for rejecting or accepting a biomaterial. This is especially true of a new biomaterial. It may, however, be possible to utilize chemical and physical-chemical determinations on extracts and, based on correlation with biological responses, establish a tolerance which, if exceeded, would fail the material. This, however, cannot and should not be done until a large battery of biological tests have been conducted and, in turn, related to the concentration and identification of the leachable ingredients. Once this has been done it may be possible to use these chemical or physical methods as quality control procedures for accepting or rejecting a biomaterial or the medical device.

Finally, there is the possibility that the presence of certain toxic chemical contaminants in the biomaterials may not be detected under the conditions of the proposed biological tests. This leads to an important point which has not been emphasized. A knowledge of the ingredients or components of a biomaterial would be of immense value to the materials toxicologist in his selection and design of both biological and analytical chemical procedures pertinent to the evaluation of specific formulations. In addition to a knowledge of the starting materials, information on the basic chemical reactions involved in the polymerization process and probable reaction products is also important. Such information would make the overall testing of a material more efficient and would provide a more reliable assessment of the safety or toxic potential of the biomaterial.

This presentation has emphasized the need for the use of a number of biological models which would help detect the presence of offending biological agents in a biomaterial. In a logical pattern of evaluation, these test procedures have been included under a preclinical testing program, referred to as "Level I Testing Program". The final development of a medical device, however, would require the device to be taken through a Level II and most likely a Level III Testing Program. In these programs, not only would the safety of the device be assessed, but equally important, the efficacy of the item would be established.

REFERENCES

1. Guess, W. L., Rosenbluth, S. A., Schmidt, B., and Autian, J., J. Pharm. Sci., 54, 156 (1965).

2. The United States of America Pharmacopeia XVIII, Mack Publishing Co., Easton, Pa., 1970, p. 926-29.

3. Autian, J., Crit. Rev. Toxicol., 2, 1 (1973).

4. Oyama, V. and Eagle, H., Proc. Soc. Exp. Biol. Med., 91, 305 (1956).

5. Lowry, O. H., Rosebrough, N. J., Farr, A. L., and Randall, R. J., J. Biol. Chem., 193, 265 (1951).

6. Turner, J. E., Lawrence, W. H., and Autian, J., J. Biomed. Mater. Res., 7, 39 (1973).

7. Magnusson, B. and Kligman, A. M., J. Invest. Dermatol., 52, 268 (1969).

8.   Draize, J. H., in Appraisal of the Safety of Chemicals in Foods, Drugs and Cosmetics, Association of Food and Drug Officials of the United States, Austin, Texas, 1959, p. 50.

SILICONE BASED RELEASE SYSTEMS

Gordon W. Duncan*, Donald R. Kalkwarf,
and Jack T. Veal

*Battelle Population Study Center, Seattle, Washington
and Battelle-Northwest Laboratories, Richland,
Washington

The pharmacologic control of fertility as presently practiced requires a substantial motivational involvement on behalf of the user and interferes with far more of the reproductive process than is necessary to achieve an acceptable level of effectiveness. A solution to both of these problems can reside in the development of delivery systems for contraceptive drugs which necessitate less overt attention by the user and/or which deliver the contraceptives more selectively to the requisite target tissue.

Use of sustained controlled release delivery systems suitable for placement within the various reproductive organs afford such an opportunity [1]. It may be anticipated that a drug delivery system of this type would:

allow for localized delivery of drug to a particular organ of interest;

provide more uniform drug concentrations at both systemic and receptor organ sites than is presently afforded by oral or parenteral dosage forms;

lower the peak systemic levels of drugs which are found after the initiation of treatment (for example, peak blood levels of equally therapeutic dosages of contraceptive steroids

205

have been found to be 100 times higher when administered by the oral route than those resulting from sustained release parenterally placed delivery systems);

improve the therapeutic spectrum of a particular drug (for example, a 25-fold increase in potency over subcutaneous or oral administration has been observed with sustained release systems);

afford contraceptive efficacy with single rather than combination drug therapy;

reduce the extent of patient involvement and/or patient-physician contact;

facilitate user acceptance and use effectiveness of the method.

Such systems, therefore, offer significant advantages for expanding the use of existing contraceptive compounds as well as an opportunity to develop new drugs from chemicals which presently are considered to have an unacceptable therapeutic ratio when administered by conventional routes of administration.

These characteristics can be achieved to some extent by manipulation of the chemical molecule itself such as by synthesis of compounds highly insoluble in body fluids (an example is Depo-Provera which affords sustained, i.e., for more than six months, blood levels following intramuscular injection) or by esterification of steroid nuclei to enhance their fat solubility and hence form depots in the body from which sustained release can subsequently occur.

An alternative approach is to incorporate drugs into biocompatible materials, either absorbable or nonabsorbable, which, when placed in the body cavity, provide prolonged controlled release of the medicament. Because of irregular release rates, minimal periods of effectiveness, and stimulation of unacceptable tissue responses to the material used in the implanted device, techniques available before the 1960s were not adequate. Of significant interest to the subsequent successful development of various systems, were the reports of Folkman and Long [2, 3] on the proposed use of silicone rubber myocardial implants and of Dzuik and Cook [4] on the release and biological effectiveness of steroids contained in silicone rubber packets and rods. This initial demon-

stration of a practical application in farm animals was followed
shortly by clinical studies of Silastic progestin-containing rods
placed subcutaneously to afford long-term contraception.

From this beginning, there has evolved a series of programs
to design devices for placement in various body cavities from
which a number of material-compound-design variations has since
emerged.

Systems Development

To date, only a few of the large number of potentially acceptable polymeric materials have been used in the fabrication of actual
delivery systems; however, a backlog of theoretical information is
accumulating, suggesting that an array of materials can be adapted
to practical clinical application. With few exceptions, almost all of
the extended clinical studies have used polydimethylsiloxane, more
commonly known as Silastic or silicone rubber. Other polymers
such as polyethylene, polypropylene, polyethylene vinyl acetate,
copolymer combinations, and hydrophilic polymers such as glycol-
methacrylate hydrogels can be used for forming simple, or multiple, or multi-layered polymer matrices. Since release rates are
influenced by the concentration, solubility and diffusivity of drug
in the polymer, an impressive array of potential materials exists
which afford a thousand-fold difference in the magnitude of the release rate for any given compound. Surface area and loading techniques can also be altered to achieve desired release rates. Generally, the objective has been to design a system which provides a
constant or zero-order release of drug for a protracted period of
time, usually one or more years. The opportunity, however,
exists to develop systems which would provide either inherently or
exogenously controlled nonlinear or rhythmic release patterns.

Contraceptive agents have also been incorporated in sustained
release systems based on the dissolution or erosion of the agent
from an implant or device such as the copper 7 IUD. Slowly dissolving copper compounds (cupric oxide, cupric carbonate) embedded in polyethylene also release copper at rates which would
enhance the contraceptive effectiveness of an otherwise inert IUD.

Development and analysis of sustained delivery systems are
generally aided by determination of release rates in vitro. A number of techniques are commonly used for such measurements. At

a minimum, the technique must provide for control of temperature
and flow of bathing medium, as these are major determinants of
release parameters. Under prescribed conditions, reliable estimates of the performance that can be expected when a particular
device is placed in vivo are obtainable. The in vitro system should
at least provide an estimate of the maximum delivery capabilities
of a certain device. Actual release rates must be studied in situ,
however, since they will be influenced by (a) the absorption by the
polymer of components of the bathing body fluids; (b) the tissue response to the device, as evidenced by encapsulation or surface deposits; (c) enhanced solubilization of the drug in tissue fluids bathing the device; and (d) local temperature variations. As might be
expected, the relationship between the observed in vivo and experimentally determined in vitro release rates depends upon the contraceptive agent, its delivery system, and the site of placement
(Fig. 1).

Systems Applications

Based upon the rapidly accumulating pool of physical/chemical
and materials information, drug delivery systems for placement
in the vagina, the cervix, the uterus, and, in the case of the male,
either in the scrotum or in some subcutaneous site are now under
development.

The first demonstrations of absorption of progestins from
Silastic devices placed in the vaginas of women utilized annular devices ranging from 50 to 90 millimeters in diameter and containing
from 50 to 2 grams of medroxyprogesterone acetate (Fig. 2). In
most cases, the devices were placed in the vagina on the fifth day
of the menstrual cycle and left in place throughout the next 21 days.
Inhibition of ovulation and evidence of systemic progestational effects were clearly demonstrated [5].

The WHO Expanded Program of Research, Development and
Research Training in Human Reproduction embarked upon the clinical evaluation of three different progestational agents, each at
several dosages. This multicentered trial is designed to identify
a progestin and a dosage level which, when released from a vaginal
device, will afford contraception without inhibiting ovulation and
without inducing an unacceptable spectrum of side effects. By
maintaining the design conformation and surface geometry constant,
and by altering the fabrication procedure and selection of polymers,

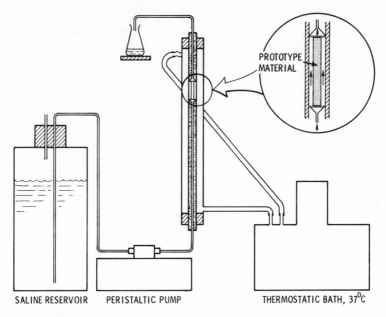

FIGURE 1. Apparatus for determination of release rates in vitro.

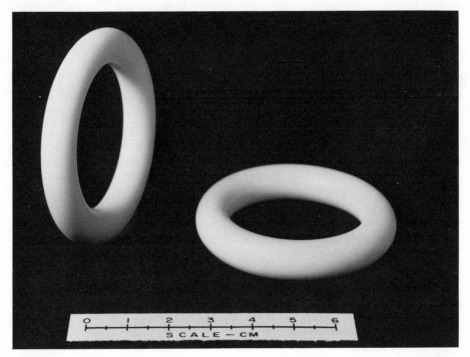

FIGURE 2. Silastic vaginal device containing 150 mg medroxyprogesterone (Provera).

it has been possible to provide daily release rates which range from a few micrograms up to several milligrams of the progestational steroids, and which can be maintained for periods up to a year. An example of the zero order release achieved with a norethindrone-loaded barrier reservoir polydimethylsiloxane device is shown in Figure 3. The device is fabricated in such manner that it has no significant burst effect, and releases ten percent of its drug during a 60-day interval.

Another approach to the delivery of contraceptive agents is the incorporation of progestins into devices designed for insertion into the uterus. While acceptable contraceptive efficacy can be achieved with certain IUDs, a satisfactory combination of efficacy and incidence of pain, bleeding, and involuntary expulsion has yet to be achieved. On the premise that local intrauterine administration of a progestin would decrease uterine sensitivity and contractility without inducing undesired systemic effects, Silastic devices containing melengestrol acetate were placed in the uteri of laboratory animals. The result supported the hypothesis and confirmed that local progestational effects on the uterus could be achieved [6]. Subsequent clinical studies demonstrated that Silastic intrauterine delivery systems can be used to deliver steroids to the human uterus in amounts sufficient to alter endometrial development

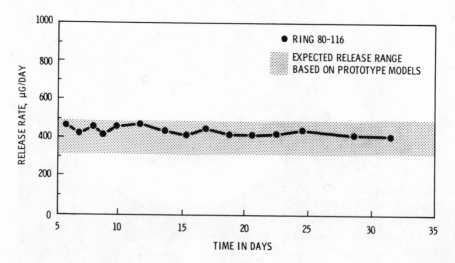

FIGURE 3. In vitro release of norethinderone from Silastic 382 vaginal rings.

without having a detectable effect on other systemic processes.
Even the effect on the endometrium was localized, there being a
gradient in response across the endometrium [7].

Scommegna, et al. examined a number of steroid-polymer
combinations as uterine delivery systems. To date, the most extensively studied preparation is Progestasert of Alza Corporation.
Designed in the shape of a T, this delivery system contains a vertical component comprised of an ethylene copolymer which serves
as a reservoir for 38 milligrams of progesterone (approximately
the amount produced by the corpus luteum each 24 hours) which,
over the course of one year, is released at the rate of 65 micrograms per day. With data accumulated from over 32 clinics
around the world, Pharriss [8] reported pregnancy rates of less
than one percent and equally acceptable incidences of expulsions
and removals for pain and bleeding. Continuation rates of 12
months were reported to approach 85 percent. This may be the
first polymeric steroidal delivery system to be marketed.

It may be parenthetically noted that, at earlier stages of development, the delivery of hemostatic and anti-inflammatory
agents at the uterine level had been examined in an attempt to provide more acceptable IUD configurations.

The cervix is also a potential site for the placement of contraceptive devices. Both WHO and the National Institute of Child
Health and Human Development are supporting studies for the development of medicated contraceptive devices to be placed in the
cervix. Medicaments being considered for inclusion in these devices are to be selected for their potential ability to alter cervical
mucous, making it hostile to sperm or giving it a direct spermi-
cidal effect.

CONCLUSION

The feasibility and value of sustained release systems for the
delivery of fertility control agents has been amply demonstrated
to date. Delivery systems for use in the vagina and the uterus are
ready for commercial introduction, and laboratory and clinical
programs seeking to improve on these accomplishments with systems designed for use in the cervix and the scrotum are in progress.

Material as well as physical chemists feel that the potential of delivery systems has only begun to be tapped. Certainly a new era of safe, effective fertility control is on the horizon, but, in addition, the development of these versatile delivery systems may provide future solutions to medical problems ranging from infertility and gynecologic disorders to those systemic disorders in females requiring subacute and chronic therapy.

REFERENCES

1. Duncan, G. W. and Kalkwarf, D. R., in Human Reproduction: Conception and Contraception, E. S. Hafez and T. N. Evans, Eds., Harper & Row, New York, 1973.

2. Folkman, G. and Long, D. M., Ann. N. Y. Acad. Sci., 111, 857 (1964).

3. Folkman, J. and Long, D. M., J. Surg. Res., 4, 139 (1964).

4. Dziuk, P. J. and Cook, B., Endocrinology, 78, 208 (1966).

5. Mishell, D. R. and Lumkin, M. E., Fertil. Steril., 21, 99 (1970).

6. Doyle, L. L. and Clewe, T. H., Amer. J. Obstet. Gynecol. 101, 564 (1968).

7. Scommegna, A., Pandya, G. N., Christ, M., Lee, A. W., and Cohen, M. R., Fertil. Steril., 21, 201 (1970).

8. Pharriss, B. B., in Intrauterine Devices: Development, Evaluation, and Program Implementation, R. G. Wheeler, G. W. Duncan, and J. J. Speidel, Eds., Academic Press, New York, 1974.

MICROCAPSULE DRUG DELIVERY SYSTEMS

Joseph A. Bakan

Research and Development Capsular Products Division,
NCR Corporation, Dayton, Ohio 45479

INTRODUCTION

Microencapsulation, a new and rapidly expanding technology
pioneered by the NCR Corporation, is receiving considerable attention both industrially and academically. Microencapsulation
is a process designed to reproducibly apply thin polymeric coatings to small particles of solids, droplets of liquid (pure or solutions), or dispersions. For the purposes of this discussion,
microencapsulation will be arbitrarily differentiated from macro-
coating techniques in that the former involves the coating of particles ranging dimensionally from several tenths of a micron to
5,000 microns in size. A unique feature of this micropackaging
technique is in the minuteness of the coated particles and their
subsequent potential usefulness in handling physiologically active
materials in a variety of dose forms.

A number of microencapsulation processes are described in
the literature, and these have been referred to as mechanical,
electrostatic or vacuum deposition and polymerization. The
processes which will be reviewed in this paper are primarily
those utilizing phase separation or coacervation techniques.

DESCRIPTION OF PROCESSES

A general outline of the batch type processes consists of a
series of three steps carried out under continuous agitation. The

1. ESTABLISHMENT OF THREE-PHASE SYSTEM

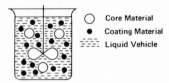

○ Core Material
● Coating Material
▭ Liquid Vehicle

2. DEPOSITION OF LIQUID-POLYMERIC COATING MATERIAL

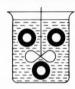

3. SOLIDIFICATION OF COATING MATERIAL

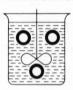

FIGURE 1. Schematic of process.

three process steps are schematically illustrated in Figure 1.

Step One of the process is the formation of three immiscible
chemical phases: a liquid manufacturing vehicle phase, a core
material phase, and a coating material phase. Step Two of the
process consists of depositing the liquid polymer coating around
the core material. This is accomplished by controlled, physical
mixing of the coating material (while liquid) and the core material
in the manufacturing vehicle. Deposition of the liquid polymer
coating around the core material occurs if the polymer is sorbed at
the interface formed between the core material and the liquid vehicle phase. This sorption phenomenon is a prerequisite to effective
coating. The continued deposition of the coating is promoted by a
reduction in the total free interfacial energy of the system brought
about by a decrease of the coating material surface area during
coalescence of the liquid polymer droplets. Step Three of the process involves rigidizing the coating, usually by thermal, crosslinking, or desolvation techniques, to form a self-sustaining entity,
i.e., a microcapsule.

Figure 2 is a photomicrograph of an encapsulated water-insoluble liquid.

Figure 3 represents a photomicrograph of an encapsulated solid.

A characteristic of microcapsules prepared by phase separation techniques is that all the particles in the batch are coated. In addition to the single particle structures shown in Figures 2 and 3, an aggregate structure can also be produced (Fig. 4) which is composed of a number of particles in cluster form. The particles in the aggregate structure need not be the same material. Figure 5 is a scanning electron micrograph of an aggregate structure.

Each particle in the aggregate structure is individually coated as is shown in the scanning electron micrograph of a sectioned aggregate capsule (Fig. 6).

CORE MATERIALS

The material to be coated should be insoluble and nonreactive with the liquid manufacturing vehicle and the coating material.

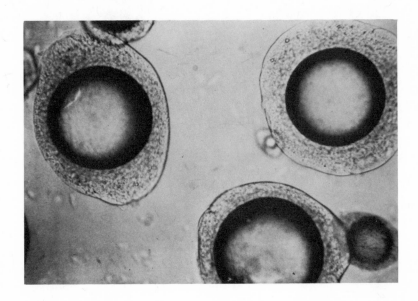

FIGURE 2. Encapsulated liquid.

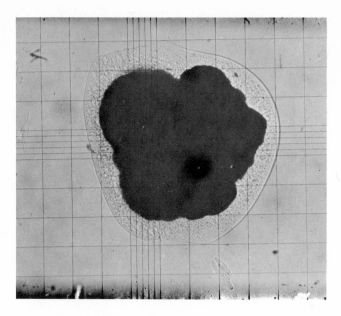

FIGURE 3.   Encapsulated solid.

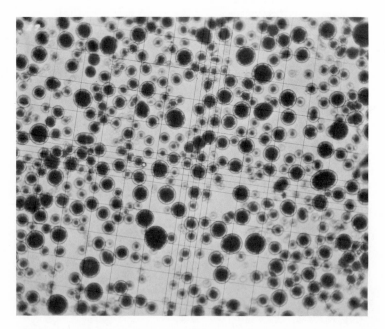

FIGURE 4.   Aggregate capsule structure.

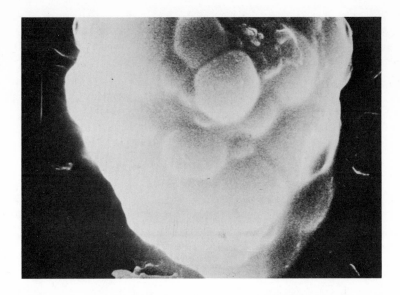

FIGURE 5. Scanning electron micrograph of aggregate capsule structure.

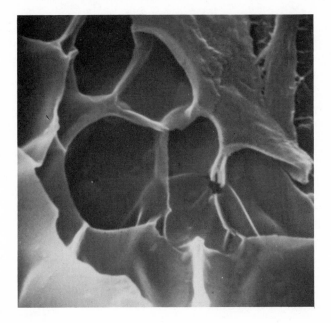

FIGURE 6. Aggregate cellular capsule structure.

Normally, water-insoluble materials are microencapsulated in aqueous vehicles, and water-soluble or organic solvent-insoluble materials are microencapsulated from organic vehicle phases. In general, water-soluble and -insoluble solids, water-insoluble liquids, solutions, and dispersions of solids in liquids can be microencapsulated. A few of the typical product classes of materials which have been microencapsulated are shown in Table I.

COATING MATERIAL

The coating material, which is basically a film-forming polymeric material, can be selected from a wide variety of natural and synthetic polymers, depending on the material to be coated and the characteristics desired in the final microcapsules. Representative coating materials are listed in Table II.

COATING WEIGHT AND CAPSULE SIZE

The amount of coating can be varied from 1% to 70% by weight. Most commercial applications normally require coating weights ranging from 3% to 30%. This corresponds to a dry film thickness from less than 1 to 200 microns, depending on the surface area of the material to be coated and other physical characteristics of the

TABLE I

TYPICAL CORE MATERIALS

Adhesives	Fuels	Perfumes
Bacteria	Growth regulators	Photographic
Blowing agents	Herbicides	agents
Catalysts	Inks	Pigments
Curing agents	Insecticides	Plasticizers
Detergents	Leavening agents	Propellants
Drugs	Metals	Solvents
Dyes	Monomers	Stabilizers
Flavors	Oils	Viruses
Foods	Paints	Vitamins

TABLE II

REPRESENTATIVE COATING MATERIALS

Aminoplasts	Gelatin-gum arabic-
Carboxymethylcellulose	ethylene maleic an-
Cellulose acetate phthalate	hydride
Ethylcellulose	Nitrocellulose
Ethylene vinyl acetate	Polyvinylalcohol
Gelatin	Propylhydroxycellulose
Gelatin-gum arabic	Shellac
Gelatin-gum arabic-vinyl	Succinylated gelatin
methylether maleic an-	Saran
hydride	Waxes

system. Figure 7 represents theoretical coating thickness versus capsule size at various core material contents. The microcapsule size can be varied from about 5 to 5,000 microns, and the structure can be of two types, a single particle structure or an aggregate structure as previously discussed.

COATING MODIFICATION

In certain product applications, it is necessary to build into the coating, characteristics not inherently present in the polymer itself. Therefore, techniques such as coloring, plasticizing, crosslinking, surface treatments, pigmentation, and multiple coatings are commonly employed in microcapsule manufacture provided that the integrity of the microencapsulated material is not altered in the modification process.

PHYSICAL FORM

The microcapsules can be isolated from their liquid manufacturing vehicle in the form of a free-flowing powder, coated on a variety of substrates, pressed or molded into briquettes, compressed into tablets, formulated as suspensions or other useful product forms.

TABLE III

STABILITY OF ENCAPSULATED LIQUIDS

Encapsulated solvent	Solvent in cap-sule %	Capsule av. size μ	Days on test	Solvent loss at 77°F 50% RH %
Benzene	85.8	500	198	0.5
Carbon tetrachloride	82.8	500	602	0.3
Chloroform	78.9	420	730	0.1
Ethylene dibromide	66.1	480	730	0.1
Hexane	70.8	35	730	0.1
Toluene	89.4	20	600	0.1
	89.9	90	600	0.1
	90.3	200	400	0.1
	90.6	480	400	0.1
	94.0	720	300	0.1
Trichloroethylene	87.2	500	400	1.0
Perchloroethylene	87.9	500	600	0.1
Xylene	90.2	500	730	0.2

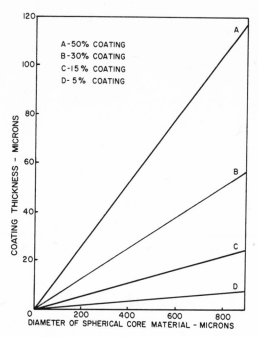

FIGURE 7. Coating thickness versus particle size at various core material contents.

STABILITY OF MICROCAPSULES

The microencapsulation of materials is of prime importance, but the microcapsules must, in turn, be stable for some period of time, in other words, have an adequate shelf life. Many volatile liquids can be microencapsulated and subsequently dried to form free-flowing powders. The data presented in Table III illustrate the liquid content of microcapsules as a function of time, showing minimal loss for the test conditions cited.

The stability of controlled release microcapsules can readily be achieved. Table IV depicts the stability and release rates of a variety of encapsulated materials under similar laboratory test conditions.

Microencapsulation can also retard the adverse effects of oxygen and water vapor on certain materials.

TABLE IV

STABILITY OF CONTROLLED RELEASE PATTERNS
OF SOLIDS HAVING VARYING DEGREES OF
WATER SOLUBILITY

Material	Time (hrs)	% Release Initial	Final	Time (mos)
Acetoaminophen	1	18	16	21
	2	35	32	
	3	49	46	
	5	69	67	
Ammonium dichromate	1	76	72	10
Acetylsalicylic acid	1	16	16	23
	2	30	30	
	3	44	45	
Sodium bicarbonate	1	9	8	30
	2	14	14	
	4	30	30	
Potassium chloride	1	74	76	25
	2	96	96	

TABLE V

SOIL EXPOSURE TEST RESULTS ON SOYBEAN OIL

Time (wks)	Peroxide value Corncobs	Microcapsules
0	2	2
1.0	2000	40
2.0	-	110
3.0	-	150
4.5	-	180
6.0	-	300

Microcapsules containing soybean oil, a highly unsaturated material subject to rapid oxidation, were compared with ground corncobs saturated with soybean oil. The data presented in Table V show the improved stability of microcapsules over a porous carrier. This stability to oxidation is measured by comparing the peroxide value when both materials are exposed on soil to ambient environmental conditions.

RELEASE PROPERTIES

Release characteristics of microencapsulated materials represent another important consideration, and a variety of mechanisms are possible.

The coating can be fractured by external forces such as pressure or by internal forces as would occur in a microcapsule having a permselective coating. The integrity of the coating can be destroyed by thermal means or by dissolution in an appropriate solvent. Release from microcapsules can be accomplished by biodegradative processes if the coatings lend themselves to such degradative mechanisms.

Another important release mechanism applicable to microcapsules is that of diffusion. If a water-soluble solid is microencapsulated in a water-insoluble film such as ethylcellulose, the contents of the microcapsule can be extracted with water. A simplified release mechanism is depicted in Figure 8.

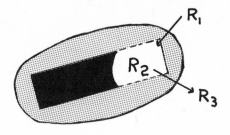

$$R_r = f(R_1, R_2, R_3)$$

FIGURE 8. Release by diffusion.

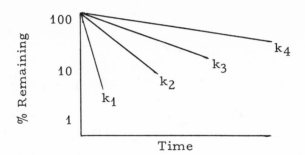

FIGURE 9. Release patterns of microencapsulated water-soluble solids by diffusion.

In the initial stage of the process, water permeates the coating. Next, an aqueous solution of the water-soluble solid is formed within the structure and this solution in turn permeates into the continuous water phase. Hence, the release rate is a function of the permeability of the film to water, the solubility of the micro-encapsulated solid, and the permeability of the film to the saturated solution. This release mechanism is independent of acidic or basic conditions, provided the film structure and the solubility of the microencapsulated material are insensitive to the varied pH conditions. R_r, the resultant release rate, can usually be described as a first-order rate process and obeys the equation $-dc/dt = kc$ where $\underline{k}$ is the velocity constant and $\underline{c}$ is the amount of material remaining in the capsule. For a specific system, the velocity constant $\underline{k}$ is inversely proportional to the film thickness. First-order release patterns are also depicted by the semilogarithmic plot in Figure 9. In practice, it has been found that, for a given microcapsular system, the velocity constant $\underline{k}$ is very reproducible.

Effective control of release properties can be achieved with materials having diverse water solubilities. Judicious selection of an appropriate coating material and variation of the coating thickness allow a spectrum of patterns to be achieved.

POTENTIAL USES OF MICROCAPSULES
FOR PHARMACEUTICALS

A variety of ethical and proprietary materials have been microencapsulated by the coacervation coating processes. A

TABLE VI

PHARMACEUTICAL CORE MATERIALS

Analgesics	Antitussives	Nutritional products
Anthelmintics	Cathartics	Potassium supplements
Antidotes	Diagnostic aids	Sedatives
Antiemetics	Diuretics	Sulfonamides
Antihistamines	Effervescents	Stimulants
Antimalarials	Enzymes	Sympathomimetics
Antimicrobials	Expectorants	Tranquilizers
Antipyretics	Hypnotics	Urinary anti-infectives
Antiseptics	Microorganisms	Vitamins
Antituberculotics	Minerals	Xanthine derivatives

representative listing of some of the generic classes of drugs which have been microencapsulated can be found in Table VI.

Microcapsules offer a variety of useful and elegant dosage forms. These include powders, hard gelatin capsules, liquid oral suspensions, hard and chewable tablets, ointments, creams, lotions, plasters, dressings and suppositories.

The potential uses of microcapsules in pharmaceuticals and related products are probably too numerous to review in detail in this discussion. Principles selected for normal consideration for pharmaceutical products include the following:

1. Converting liquids to solids
2. Separating reactive materials
3. Taste masking of bitter drugs
4. Prolonged action medicaments

In the following paragraphs, the above contributions of microcapsules will be discussed.

Converting Liquids to Solids

Scientists have noted that selected organic compounds, in the thermal transformation from solid to liquid state, passed through

TABLE VII

CLASSIFICATION OF THERMOTROPIC LIQUID
CRYSTALS BASED ON MICROSCOPIC AND
X-RAY STUDIES*

1. Nematic
        Classical nematic
        Twisted nematic or cholesteric
        Cybotactic nematic
        Skewed cybotactic nematic

2. Smectic
        Eight polymorphic forms, identified
        as Smectic A, B, C, D, E, F, G,
        and H

*Chem. Technol., Jan., 1973.

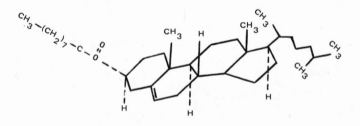

FIGURE 10.   Cholesteryl nonanoate.

an intermediate phase which exhibited the anisotropic (having optical direction) properties of crystalline solids. The term "liquid crystal state" has been coined to describe this ordered phenomenon. The liquid crystal state or mesophase has been scientifically classified into distinct categories based on the mode of penetration (thermotropic or lyotropic) into the liquid crystalline region as well as the ordering and degree of spatial arrangement of the molecules in the mass of the material. Table VII depicts the classification of thermotropic liquid crystal systems which will be discussed here.

The normal phase transition occurring with these materials follows the general path:

Crystalline ——→ Liquid crystal state ——→ Isotropic liquid
solid   (anisotropic liquid)   (without optical
                                             direction)

In thermotropic-type liquid crystals, this phase transition is induced by temperature change.

NCR has been most interested in thermotropic liquid crystals, more specifically, the twisted nematic or cholesteric materials which will be elaborated upon here.

Molecules which traverse this thermotropic liquid crystalline state are normally long and rod-shaped, and are oriented in planar configurations in the mass of the material. A typical organic compound which possesses the molecular geometry required for forming a liquid crystal mesophase, namely, cholesterylnonanoate is represented in Figure 10.

Cholesteric or twisted nematic structure is depicted in Figure 11.

Cholesterol esters, which traverse the cholesteric state, exhibit anisotropic optical properties of crystalline solids. As a result of the unique structure of the phase, iridescent colors are observed in the material when they are illuminated with white light at a given temperature.

A cholesteric liquid crystal system, when formulated properly, responds to changes in temperature by sequentially passing through

PROBABLE ORGANIZATION
OF CHOLESTERIC PHASE

CHOLESTERIC LC
MESOPHASE

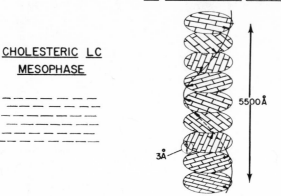

FIGURE 11. Cholesteric liquid crystals have a readily alterable
helical structure.

the complete visual spectrum - red through violet - in fractions of
degrees, or multidegrees, depending on the cholesterol esters
comprising the formulation. This color phenomenon is reversible
and has been reported to function over a temperature range of
-20°C to 250°C.

Colors scattered by liquid crystals represent only a fraction
of the incident light. The remaining portion of the incident light
is transmitted by the liquid crystals.

An absorptive black background, therefore, is needed to prevent reflection of the transmitted light, thereby enhancing the purity or resolution of the scattered colors or wavelengths reflected
by the liquid crystal system.

Encapsulated liquid crystal (ELC) material systems are a new
concept in the field of thermally sensitive compounds. Through
the use of this modern concept in packaging labile materials, a
new vista of medical applications, heretofore not considered, becomes potentially feasible. These tiny packages, 2-50 microns
in diameter, offer several major advantages:

1. Convert the liquid crystal system to a pseudo-solid, providing ease of handling, application, and use.

2. Provide longer shelf life by minimizing surface contamination and giving protection from ultra-violet light.

ELCs have been produced in a variety of forms. The capsules can be supplied as a water-based slurry suitable for application by conventional coating, brushing, or spraying.

The ELCs can also be supplied in the form of coatings on a variety of substrates. Standard substrates include various paper stocks and Mylar. The substrates normally used are black or they can be coated with an absorptive black background. The ELC can also be coated without an absorptive black background.

Standard ELC materials are available in three series as shown in Table VIII.

TABLE VIII

STANDARD ELC PRODUCTS (APPROXIMATE COLORPLAY RANGE)

Series	Colorplay	Temperature range, °C
S (Sensitive)	$1.5 \pm 0.5°C$ (*)	15 - 70
R (Regular)	$3.5 \pm 1.0°C$ (**)	15 - 55
W (Wide)	$6.0 \pm 2.0°C$ (**)	0 - 45

(*) Start of red to end of blue
(**) Start of red to start of blue

Medical diagnostic applications of encapsulated liquid crystals which are now under investigation and show favorable results inclued the following:

1. Normal vascular physiology

2. Diseased vascular states
    Pulmonary vascular disease
    Cardiac vascular disease
    Peripheral vascular disease
    Breast malignancies
    Other tumors

3. Effects of nerve-blocking drugs upon circulation

4. Location of the placental attachment in obstetrics

Separation of Incompatibles

Separation or isolation of reactive materials can readily be accomplished through microencapsulation as all particles subjected to the process are completely coated. Figure 12 shows the salicylic acid buildup with time for a mixture of propoxyphene hydrochloride aspirin as well as the aspirin control. The microencapsulation of both materials produced a substantially more stable mixture.

Taste Masking of Bitter Drugs

The taste masking of bitter drugs can be accomplished in chewable tablet form.

Water-soluble or partially water-soluble solids can be encapsulated in water-insoluble films. A bitter-tasting drug such as acetyl p-aminophenol (APAP) can be coated to produce a dry, free-flowing APAP which is effectively taste-masked. These capsules can be formulated with appropriate excipients into a chewable tablet dosage form.

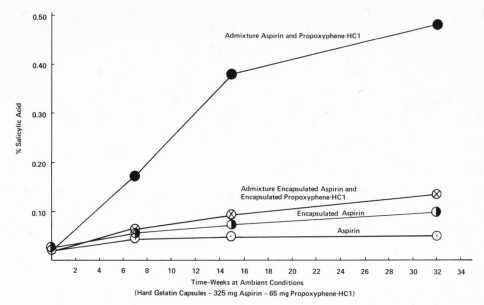

FIGURE 12. Separation of incompatibles.

TABLE IX

TASTE-MASKED CHEWABLE APAP TABLETS

1. ENCAPSULATED APAP
      CORE MATERIAL : N-ACETYL-P-AMINO PHENOL
      COATING : CELLULOSIC-WAX
      APAP CONTENT : 91%
      PARTICLE SIZE : -100 MESH
      p-AMINOPHENOL CONTENT : 0.01%
      RESIDUAL SOLVENT : <50 ppm.

2. TABLETED CAPSULAR APAP
      TABLET WEIGHT : 755 mg.
      APAP CONTENT : 327 mg.
      DISINTEGRATION TIME : 15 MIN.
         (ROTATING BOTTLE)
      IN VITRO RELEASE : 10 MIN. - 56 %
                          30 MIN. - 89%
         (GERSHBERG STOLL, 37°C -1.2 pH)

3. TABLET BASE
      MANNITOL   TALC
      AVICEL   MAGNESIUM STEARATE
      CORN STARCH   SACCHARIN
      SODIUM CYCLAMATE   GUM GUAR
      PEPPERMINT FLAVOR   MINT-SPICE FLAVOR

Normally, for taste masking purposes, the availability of the drug must not be altered. The objective of encapsulation is to provide as much protection as possible without inhibiting the availability of the drug.

Table IX depicts the microcapsule, tablet, and base properties of a typical taste-masked chewable tablet.

Prolonged Action Medicaments

Another significant application of microencapsulation is the contribution it can make in the prolonged action or sustained release field.

Not all drugs, of course, are amenable to prolonged action or sustained release dosage forms. Among the assumptions for drug candidates amenable to sustained or prolonged action, are uniform absorption of the drug in the gastrointestinal system, ready availability of the drug at the absorption sites, patient variances, uniform time constants, pH effects, etc. Even considering these and other seemingly narrow theoretical restrictions, a large number of candidates still exist.

Microencapsulation can contribute significantly in this area in that the release mechanism of a water-soluble or partially water-soluble drug from a capsule can be based on diffusion principles. Coatings can be applied to small solid particles that are insoluble in the gastrointestinal tract and are unaffected by enzymes and pH, thus limiting the in vivo variability of the drug release. The fact that microcapsules are very small assists in the uniform distribution of the drug reservoir in the gastrointestinal tract. Release of the medicaments from microcapsules is accomplished by diffusion principles.

By starting with a given in vitro release pattern for encapsulated aspirin (Fig. 13), variations in the bioavailability of the encapsulated form of the drug can be demonstrated. By varying the in vitro patterns, the in vivo responses can obviously be changed, and thus the therapeutic effectiveness of the material can potentially be extended.

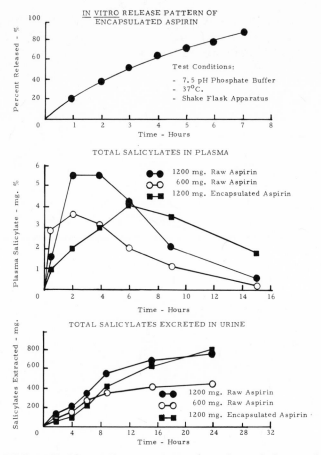

FIGURE 13.   Microencapsulated aspirin study.

SUMMARY

In summation, it is believed that microencapsulation offers a technical base from which many new and innovative products can be developed for the pharmaceutical industry because of the following attributes of microencapsulation:

1. Ability to apply continuous coatings to all products
2. Ability to coat small and large particles
3. Ability to coat liquids and solids
4. Reproducible coating properties, that is, thickness, permeability control, active content, etc.
5. Proven adaptability to sustained production on a tonnage scale.

As one works in the field of microencapsulation, the many possibilities present themselves for the creative individual to develop new and useful products, heretofore considered impossible without microcapsules.

ACKNOWLEDGEMENTS

The author would like to express his appreciation to his colleagues at the NCR Corporation whose research contributed to this review paper.

REFERENCES

1. Brynko, C., U. S. Patent 2,969,330 (1961).

2. Brynko, C., Bakan, J. A., Miller, R. E., and Scarpelli, J. A., U. S. Patent 3,341,466 (1967).

3. Brynko, C., Olderman, G., U. S. Patent 3,516,943 (1970).

4. Green, B. K., U. S. Patent 2,730,456 (1956).

5. Green, B. K., et al., U. S. Patent 2,870,457 (1959).

6. Herbig, J. A., in Encyclopedia of Chemical Technology, 2nd ed, R. E. Kirk and D. F. Othmer, Eds., Interscience Publishers, John Wiley and Sons, New York, 1967, Vol. 13, p. 436.

7. Herbig, J. A., and Hanny, J. F., U. S. Patent 3,161,602 (1964).

8. Heistand, E. N., Wagner, J. G., and Knoechel, E. L., U. S. Patent 3,242,051 (1966).

9. Miller, R. E., and Anderson, J. L., U. S. Patent 3,155,590 (1964).

10. Powell, T. C., Steinle, M. E., and Yoncoski, R. A., U. S. Patent 3,415,758 (1968).

11.   The Condensed Chemical Dictionary, 4th ed, Reinhold
      Publishing Co., New York, 1950, p. 178.

12.   Bakan, J. A., and Anderson, J. L., in The Theory and
      Practice of Industrial Pharmacy, L. Lachman, H. Liberman,
      and J. Kanig, Eds., Lea & Febiger, Philadelphia, Pa.,
      1970, p. 384.

13.   Bakan, J. A., presented at Land O'Lakes Industrial
      Pharmaceutical Conference, June, 1966.

14.   Bakan, J. A., presented at Eastern Regional IPT Section,
      Academy of Pharmaceutical Sciences, Philadelphia, Pa.
      October, 1968.

15.   Bell, S. A., Berdick, M., and Holliday, W. M., J. New
      Drugs, 6, September-October, 1966.

16.   Chameleon Compounds, Science News, September, 1968.

17.   Churchill, D., Cartmell, J., Miller, R., British Patent
      1, 138, 590 (1969).

18.   Encapsulated Liquid Crystals, NCR Brochure.

19.   Gardner, G. L., presented at the Symposium on Pharma-
      ceutical Processing, 58th Annual Meeting, Philadelphia, Pa.,
      December, 1965.

20.   Tricoire, J., Presse Med., 78, 2481 (1970).

21.   Potanin, C., presented at the 19th Annual Scientific Session
      of the American College of Cardiology, New Orleans, La.,
      February-March, 1970.

22.   Potanin, C., Russell, R. O., Jr., Rackley, C. E., and
      Dodge, H. T., Lancet, 2, 663 (1969).

23.   Tricoire, J., Mariel, L., Amiel, J. P., et al., Presse
      Med., 78, 2483 (1970).

24.   Bakan, J. A. and Sloan, F. D., Drug Cosmet. Ind., 110,
      34 (1972).

DRUG DELIVERY SYSTEMS: DESIGN CRITERIA

Donald R. Cowsar

Southern Research Institute
Birmingham, Alabama

In the context of the current state of the art, a controlled release drug delivery system is a combination of drug and excipient, commonly a polymeric material, arranged to allow delivery of the drug to the target at controlled rates over a specified time. The polymeric material may be either biodegradable or nonbiodegradable, and the drug may be released by diffusion of the drug through the encapsulating polymer matrix, by erosion of the polymer matrix, by a combination of diffusion and erosion, or by an alternative physical phenomenon such as capillary flow through wicks of fluid-filled devices and displacement by physiological fluids. The physical forms of the controlled release doses can vary considerably and currently include macrocapsules or pellets that are implanted via incision or trocar, microcapsules or microparticles that are injected via a syringe; envelopes, films, or laminates that are placed in the cul-de-sac of the eye or in the oral cavity, or are implanted subcutaneously; various ring- and T-shaped intravaginal and intrauterine devices; and bandages for topical and transdermal delivery.

BASIC PRINCIPLES

Pharmaceutical companies expend vast efforts and funds synthesizing, screening, and testing new drugs. However, once a promising compound has been identified, considerably less effort is usually spent developing the delivery system, i.e., the final dosage form. Standard criteria are usually followed to determine the best conventional route of administration, the unit dose, the drug half-life, and the most effective or convenient dosage schedule. Drugs are usually administered orally or via injection, often at a site remote from the target. Figure 1 shows schematically the delivery of drugs by conventional techniques. Route 1 in the figure illustrates oral administration. In this case, the drug first enters the digestive tract having a volume, V_1. Here the drug becomes diluted. Over a period of time, the drug either diffuses into the systemic circulation having a volume, V_2, or is removed from V_1 via excretion or chemical deactivation. In the figure, K_r is the rate constant for removal of the drug from V_1. As the drug enters V_2 it becomes further diluted as it is distributed to the various organs, O, at least one of which is the target for the drug. The action of the drug on organs other than the target may result in undesirable side effects. Finally, the drug is metabolized or otherwise irreversibly removed from V_2 at a rate governed by the removal rate constant, $k_r^!$. Route 2 in the figure illustrates a more direct application such as by intravenous or intramuscular injection. The first reservoir, V_1, is circumvented, but side effects resulting from drug in V_2 affecting nontarget organs can still occur.

When drugs are delivered by one of these conventional routes, the drug level and duration of bioavailability cannot be controlled independently. Only the size and frequency of the dose can be manipulated. The rate of removal of drug from the body is usually considered to be an "uncontrollable" parameter. At best, the removal of drug can be described by typical reaction kinetics, with most biological removal systems being first-order in drug concentration.

Figure 2 schematically shows the concept of controlled delivery of drugs. This figure has some obvious similarities with the first figure. For controlled delivery, however, the delivery rate constants, k_d, are important parts of the scheme. For delivery via "Route 1", a controlled release formulation of the drug is administered to the total systemic biological environment by injection or implantation. The dosage form is a drug reservoir that protects the stored drug from removal mechanisms and delivers the drug to the biological reservoir, V_2, at a predetermined (programmed) rate, k_d. Only the release drug is subject to removal via metabolism and excretion. For delivery via "Route 2", the controlled release formulation is positioned in the biological environment in close proximity to the target to permit delivery of

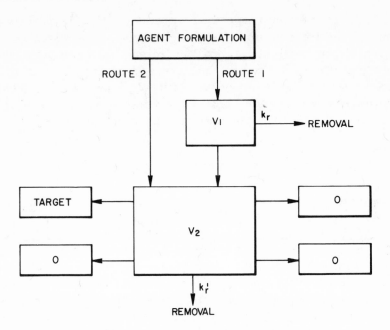

FIGURE 1. Conventional drug delivery.

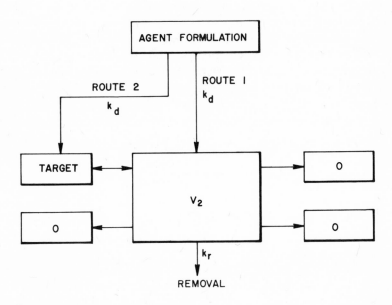

FIGURE 2. Controlled release delivery of drugs.

the drug directly to the target at a rate, k_d. For drug delivery
via Route 1 the total volume, V_2, of the systemic circulation (or
the patient's body weight), is still an important variable since,
like in conventional delivery, the released drug is diluted by this
V_2 factor. For drug delivery via Route 2, however, very little
dilution occurs and, hence, only very small amounts of drug are
required to produce the optimum biological response.

SPECIFIC DESIGN CRITERIA

Not all drugs are amenable to administration by controlled
delivery formulations. Candidate drugs must be potent and stable
to storage at physiological temperatures for long periods. Given,
however, that one has a potent drug that is difficult to administer
by conventional means, either because it requires hospitalization
of the patient for frequent injections which is expensive or because
it can produce serious side effects when the bioavailability is not
controlled at some optimum level, then the design of a controlled
delivery dosage form should be considered.

The first design parameter that should be considered is the
drug release rate that the system should provide. This can usually
be approximated from pharmacokinetic data obtained by conventional means. If the physiological half-life of the drug is known,
one can usually apply first-order removal rate kinetics to calculate
an approximate delivery rate required to maintain optimum bioavailability. The first order rate law states that the instantaneous
rate of removal is proportional to the amount of drug present. If
M/V_2 is the concentration of drug present, the rate of removal,
$\dfrac{d(M/V_2)}{dt}$, of drug can be expressed as

$$\frac{d(M/V_2)}{dt} = k_r(M/V_2) \tag{1}$$

where k_r is the rate constant for removal. The integrated solution to Eq. 1 is

$$\ln M/M_o = k_r t \tag{2}$$

where M_o is the amount present at $t = 0$. The rate of removal
is usually expressed as the drug half-life, $t_{1/2}$. The half-life is

related to the first-order rate constant for removal as follows:

$$\ln 2 = k_r t_{1/2} \tag{3}$$

or

$$k_r = \ln 2/t_{1/2} = 0.693/t \tag{4}$$

If the controlled delivery system is being designed to deliver the drug at a constant rate (zero-order kinetics), the delivery rate can be expressed mathematically as

$$\frac{d(M/V_2)}{dt} = k_d \tag{5}$$

If drug removal follows first-order kinetics then the level of drug availability will be constant when the rate of delivery equals the rate of removal, or when

$$k_d = k_r \, M/V_2 \tag{6}$$

or

$$k_d = 0.693/t_{1/2}(M/V_2) \tag{7}$$

For example, if the drug has a half-life of six hours and the optimum systemic level of bioavailability is 6 μg/kg, then a controlled release dosage form for a 75 kg patient should deliver the drug at 52 μg/hr or 1.2 mg/day. A dosage form that would have a duration of activity of 30 days would have to contain at least 36 mg of drug. On the other hand, if the dosage form is designed to deliver the drug directly to the target, e.g., an IUD that releases a contraceptive steroid directly to the female reproductive organs, the dilution factor, V_2, becomes insignificant and a release rate of perhaps 3 μg/hr or less would be sufficient. In this case a delivery system containing 36 mg of drug could be effective for about 16 months.

Once estimates have been made of the desired rate and duration of release, the dosage form designer must consider a myriad of other design parameters including the following:

The desired site or route of administration of the controlled release dose is perhaps most important. As mentioned earlier, a delivery system placed in close proximity to the target organ is usually most desirable. The delivery of ophthalmic preparations directly to the eye via a device such as the new product, Ocusert, of Alza Corp., and the delivery of contraceptive steroids directly to the female reproductive organs via devices such as the Alza Progestasert IUD or the intravaginal rings discussed earlier take into account this advantage. The Ocusert, a pilocarpine ocular delivery system for the treatment of glaucoma, delivers the drug to the eye from a membrane-laminate placed under the lower eyelid. Delivery occurs at a nearly constant rate (20 to 40 µg/hr, depending upon the membrane) for a period of one week. The Progestasert, an intrauterine progesterone delivery system for contraceptive use, delivers progesterone to the uterine lumen at an essentially constant rate of 65 µg/day for a period of more than one year. My group at Southern Research Institute is currently developing an intraoral delivery system for fluoride.* When the site of administration of the controlled release dose is a convenient body cavity, the polymeric excipient can usually be easily retrieved once the drug has been released. This, in turn, means that the excipient can be selected from a relatively large number of biocompatible, nonbiodegradable polymers.

Controlled release dosage forms can be injected or implanted near the target or in highly vascularized tissues. Some of the earliest work with controlled release systems involved subcutaneous implants of silicone rubber-encapsulated steroids and pacemaker drugs. The limitation of implants of course is that spent devices of nonbiodegradable material must be retrieved and this usually means surgical removal. The use of biodegradable polymeric excipients eliminates the problem of removal, but the number of currently known biodegradable (absorbable) polymers is small. Homopolymeric and copolymeric hydroxyacetic acid esters, e.g., polyglycolic acid and polylactic acid, and natural polymers such as collagen, starch, and chitin are being investigated as biodegradable excipients for implantable delivery systems.

The mechanisms and rates of drug release from controlled delivery systems are the key design considerations that ultimately separate controlled release from slow release, a much older and well recognized concept from which the new science is emerging. Slow release formulations are so-called because they contain several times the normal single dose and they provide for replacement of agent at some rate which gives a measurable increase in the

*Funded by the National Institute of Dental Research.

length of time of activity. Slow release can be achieved by a number of methods including the use of slowly dissolving coatings, of complexes, and of derivatives having reduced solubility. In general, these mechanisms are sensitive to changes in the biological environment to which they are exposed. In controlled release systems, on the other hand, the release rate is determined by the physicochemical properties of the system itself.

Typically, controlled delivery systems are designed to release the polymer-encapsulated drug at a constant or slowly declining rate by erosion of the polymer or by membrane-moderated Fickian diffusion. To release drug by erosion, the polymeric excipient need not be permeable to the drug but it must degrade at an appropriate rate and the degradation products must be completely and harmlessly metabolized. To release agent by diffusion, the polymeric excipient must be permeable to the drug, and its permeability must not be adversely affected by its environment.

Although the size and shape of controlled release systems can vary from micro- and macro-particles and -spheres to discs, rods, films and filaments, most current erodible and diffusion-controlled formulations are of two basic designs: (1) those in which the drug forms a core surrounded by the polymeric excipient, and (2) those in which the drug is dispersed (or sometimes dissolved) in the polymer matrix. The first type is usually called a "reservoir" system, and the second type is usually called a "monolithic" system. A good review of the mechanisms and rates of drug release via diffusion from reservoir and monolithic devices is now available [1]. In general, for diffusion-type reservoir systems, release rate can be constant (zero-order), providing the system is designed to maintain unit thermodynamic activity immediately inside the rate-limiting membrane. Unit activity is achieved when a saturated solution with excess solid phase is present, or a pure liquid phase or solid phase is present within the lumen of the system. For diffusion-type monolithic systems with excess dispersed drug, the release rate is proportional to the square root of the drug loading and the rate slowly decreases according to the square-root-of-time rate law.

Finally, the ability of the dosage form to be fabricated (ultimately mass production) must be taken into account. Most common polymeric materials are fabricated into various shapes by thermoforming (molding or extrusion) processes. Temperatures ranging from 150 to 300°C are commonly employed. Some polymer systems require free radical catalysts as well as heat for vulcanization.

When polymer solutions are used for coatings and film making, the solvents used are frequently either exotic, e.g., hexafluoroacetone sesquihydrate and hexafluoroisopropanol, or reactive, e.g., formic acid, aqueous sodium hydroxide, and mixed phenols. If one considers formulating drugs in microcapsules or monolithic films or polymeric excipients that are traditionally fabricated under conditions that are not compatible with the agents, considerable effort is often required to find alternative fabrication techniques. One reason that silicone rubber emerged early as the most important material in this new field of controlled release is its ease of fabrication. A number of new materials are under investigation that offer specific advantages of ease of fabrication, optimum release characteristics, and in some cases, biodegradability.

CONCLUSIONS

The designers of controlled delivery dosage forms must have an unusually high degree of understanding of a variety of design parameters and system variables in order to develop the desired degree of control. Because of the magnitude and interdisciplinary nature of the effort, the task cannot be undertaken lightly, but must be fully justified by the increased value of the system. Dosage form design cannot be merely appended to an extensive drug development program. In fact, in the context of current FDA regulations, all drug excipient controlled delivery formulations are considered new drugs and must be subjected to extensive safety and efficacy evaluations even if the components have been separately approved. Nevertheless, the new technology opens up novel approaches to overcoming inefficient delivery of drugs, which has long been a barrier to the fuller utilization of a number of important pharmaceutical compounds.

REFERENCE

1.   Tanquary, A. C. and Lacey, R. E., Eds., in Controlled Release of Biologically Active Agents, Adv. Exp. Med. Biol. 47, 1974.

CONTROLLED RELEASE OF BIOLOGICALLY ACTIVE AGENTS

Seymour Yolles

Department of Chemistry, University of Delaware
Newark, Delaware 19711

The development of injectable systems for sustained delivery
of drugs at a controlled rate has been the object of various publications. In 1946, a patent [1] was issued claiming pellets consisting of dispersions of a desiccated hormone in waxy media as
a new system for a slow and prolonged release of active materials.
Substitution of the waxy media as matrices by silicones for fertility control was reported by other investigators [2, 3, 4, 5]. A
recent innovation is the use of biodegradable polymers such as
polylactic acid (PLA), which will also assure a complete delivery
of the drug [6].

Several papers have been published dealing with factors influencing the release of a drug from waxy granular matrices [7]
and from methylacrylate-methylmethacrylate copolymers [8]. In
addition, various investigators have presented mathematical approaches to describe the migration of a drug through solid polymer matrices of various shapes [5, 9, 10, 11].

Composites of drugs and polymeric matrices are at present
under intense investigation as fertility control agents [3, 4, 5, 12],
narcotic antagonists [6, 13, 14], anticancer agents [15], weight-
gaining agents for beef cattle [16] and for the treatment of glaucoma [17] and ulcers [18].

The system for sustained delivery of drugs investigated by
this laboratory comprises incorporating a drug in a polymeric

245

matrix, shaping the composite into a convenient form such as
films, pellets or chips, and then implanting the structure into the
body tissue of animals by surgery or hypodermic injection. The
drug diffuses continuously from the interior of the polymeric composite to the outer surface, where it is mechanically swept away
by body fluids surrounding the structure. The mechanism of migration through the polymer is that of diffusion and the thermodynamic driving force is the concentration gradient [9, 10].

Previous papers [6, 19] from this laboratory have dealt with
the influence of the following factors on the release of cyclazocine
(2-cyclopropylmethyl-2'-hydroxy-5,9-dimethyl-6,7-benzomorphan;
Structure I, Fig. 1): (a) nature of the polymer, polyethylene and
polylactic acid, (b) molecular weight of the polymer and (c) form
of the composites, films and particles.

We report in this paper the results of recent investigations
concerning (1) release rates of two new narcotic antagonists,
naloxone (17-allyl-4,5-a-epoxy-3,14-dihydroxymorphinan-6-one, II,

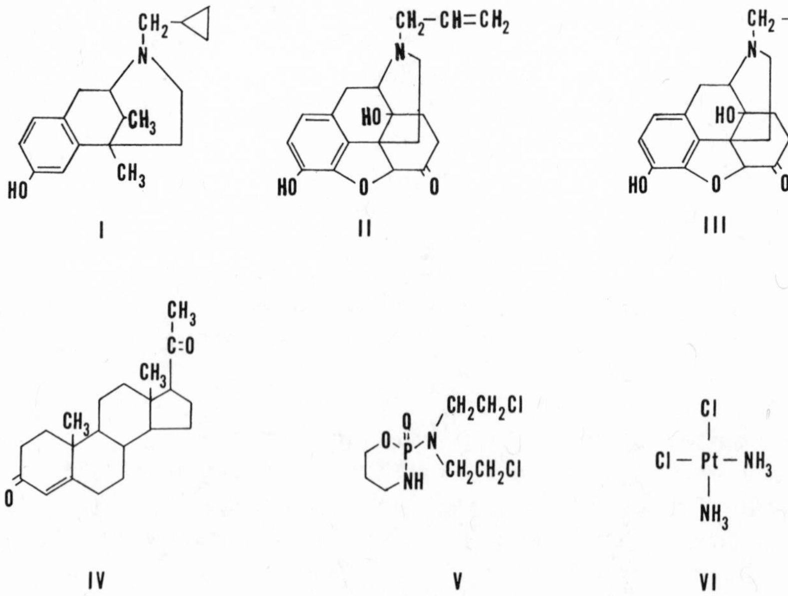

FIGURE 1

and naltrexone (17-cyclopropylmethyl-4, 5-α-epoxy-3, 4-dihydroxy-morphinan-6-one, III), of a fertility control drug, progesterone (Δ^4-pregnene-3, 20-dione, IV) and of two potent anticancer agents, cytoxan (2-[bis(2-chloroethyl)amino] tetrahydro-2H-1, 3, 2-oxaza-phosphorine-2-oxide, V) and cis-dichlorodiammineplatinum (II) (formula VI) and (2) influence of the particle size of naltrexone composites and of the concentration of naltrexone in composites on the release rates. The chemical structures of these compounds are also shown in Figure 1.

Composites were prepared by melt-pressing into sheets a mixture of drug (in most cases partially tritiated), polymer (poly-ethylene or polylactic acid) and a plasticizer (tributyl citrate). Temperatures varying between 140°C and 165°C and a pressure of one metric ton load for 10 seconds were generally used. Compos-ites containing 20% and 35% of drug were investigated. Films so ob-tained were used as such, in samples of 1-2 sq cm, or were re-duced to small particles, and fractions of average sizes 100, 200, 350 and 600 microns were collected. Specific radioactivities of the composites were determined by combustion of the polymer matrices and radioassaying the water trapped in a Tricarb Oxi-dizer System. For the anticancer composites, the amount of drug in the polymer was determined by quantitative analysis, e.g., atomic absorption spectroscopy.

Efficacy of these composites was determined by measuring the release rates of the drug in vivo (rats or rabbits) and in vitro and by the physiological responses in rats, dogs, monkeys, and mice.

In experiments in vivo, the delivery rates of the drug were determined by surgically implanting or hypodermically injecting the composites into the animals and measuring at fixed intervals of time the radioactivity of urine or analyzing the amount of drug in urine. In several cases, at the end of the experiment, the composites were collected from the sacrificed animal and the amount of drug left in the composite was determined.

In experiments in vitro, the delivery rates were determined by extracting samples of composites with tepid water (29°C ± 3°C) in a modified Raab extractor [6] and measuring the amount of drug in the extracted aqueous solution at fixed intervals of time.

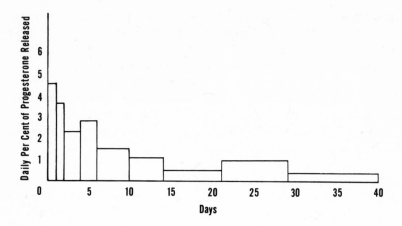

FIGURE 2

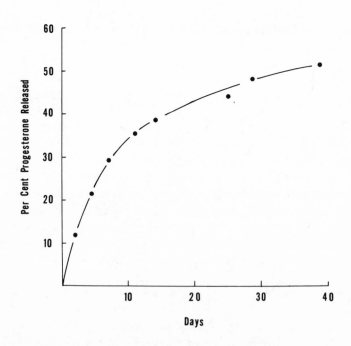

FIGURE 3

The physiological response in animals was investigated with naltrexone composites by measuring the duration of morphine antagonist activity.

FERTILITY CONTROL DRUG COMPOSITES

The in vivo release of progesterone from a polyethylene matrix in film form was determined by implanting the film into rabbits and monitoring the radioactivity of the urine. The results obtained are reported in Figures 2 and 3. The daily amounts of progesterone released after reaching a maximum during the first two to six days from implantation, decreased in the following five days, then remained relatively constant for the duration of the test.

The cumulative amount of drug released in urine during the 39-day test period was 51% of the administered dose. However, the determination of drug present in the composite at the end of a 60-day test showed that the amount of drug released was higher, averaging 80% of the dose.

Thus, the feasibility of sustained delivery of fertility control drugs has been demonstrated.

NARCOTIC ANTAGONIST COMPOSITES

Parallel in vivo and in vitro tests have been performed to determine the release rates of cyclazocine, naloxone and naltrexone from PLA composites in particle form and to investigate the influence of the particle size of the composites and of the concentration of the drug in the composites on the release rates.

The results of the in vivo and in vitro release of cyclazocine from composites containing 20% drug are reported in Figure 4. In the in vivo tests, the cumulative amount of cyclazocine excreted in urine within 54 days was 20% of the administered dose. The in vitro delivery rate of cyclazocine is more rapid than in vivo, as might be expected, due to the large excess of extractant present in the in vitro tests.

The in vitro and in vivo release rates of naloxone and naltrexone from composites containing 20% drug are reported in

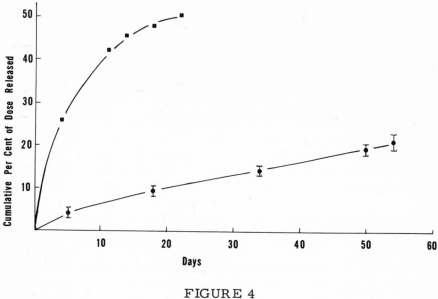

FIGURE 4

Figures 5 and 6, respectively. The results of the in vivo tests are comparable to those obtained with cyclazocine. However, in the case of naltrexone, the release rate slows down after 35 days from implantation.

The parallel experiments in vitro showed that the delivery rates of cyclazocine and naltrexone are considerably faster than in vivo, whereas that of naloxone is similar to that found in vivo, within experimental errors. This behavior of naloxone in comparison with the other two drugs could be due to differences in the physical makeup of the composites, caused by different melting points and solubilities of these drugs in the polymer.

Influence of Particle Size on Release Rates

The influence of the particle size of the composites on the release rates of the narcotic antagonists was studied with composites of 350 and 600 microns containing naloxone and with composites of 100, 200, 350 and 600 microns containing naltrexone. The particle size shows only a moderate influence on the release rate of naloxone (Fig. 7).

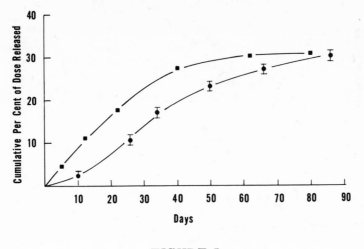

FIGURE 5

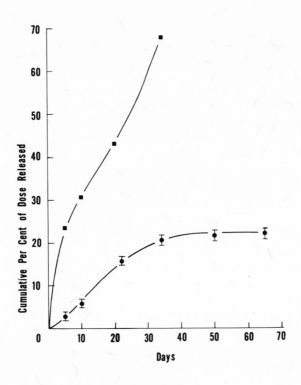

FIGURE 6

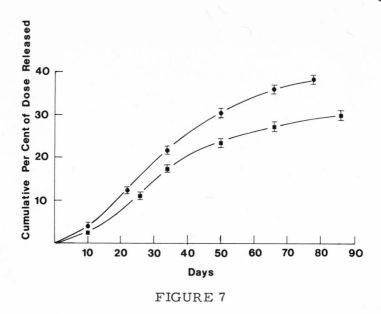

FIGURE 7

A significant difference in the amounts of drug released between large (600 microns) and small (100-350 microns) particles
was observed in in vivo tests with naltrexone (Fig. 7), the smaller
particles releasing at a faster rate than the larger. A small
difference, however, was observed for particles varying in size
between 100 and 350 microns. All the sizes investigated, 100-
600 microns, are in the usable range for injection as suspensions
in carboxymethyl (CM) cellulose.

Influence of Concentration of Drug in Composites on the Release Rates

Composites of tritiated naltrexone-PLA containing 20 and 35%
of naltrexone have been injected as suspensions of particles (600
microns) into rats and the amounts of naltrexone excreted in urine
measured.

The total cumulative amounts of naltrexone excreted over a
period of 54 days were 21. 0 and 11. 0% of the administered dose,
respectively (Fig. 9), indicating that a considerable amount of
drug was not recovered in urinary excretion. When the above
amount of naltrexone excreted was plotted as mg vs time (Fig. 10),

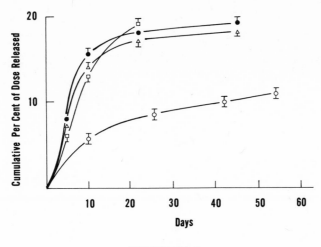

FIGURE 8

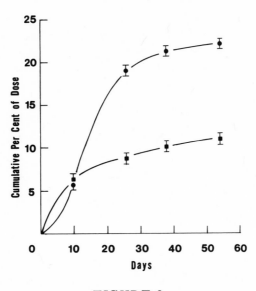

FIGURE 9

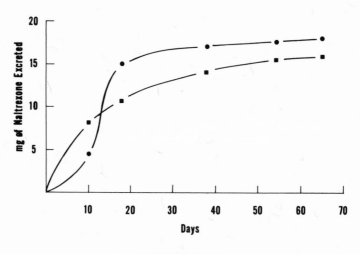

FIGURE 10

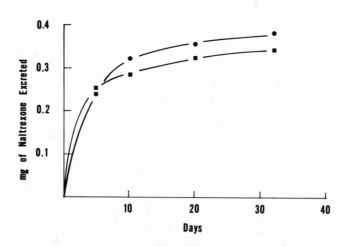

FIGURE 11

the curves showed that the amount of drug excreted is independent of the concentration of the drug in the composites. It appear from the shapes of these curves that the animal is able to process and eliminate in the urine only a certain amount of drug, a ceiling above which more drug is not excreted.

These data on the release of naltrexone are substantiated by experiments performed by injecting different amounts of tritiated naltrexone hydrochloride, 1.6 and 3.2 mg/kg, into rats as solutions in normal saline, and measuring the radioactivity of the urinary excretion. At the end of a 32-day experiment, the amount of naltrexone found in the urine was 0.34 mg when 1.6 mg/kg of naltrexone was injected and 0.38 mg when 3.2 mg/kg was injected (Fig. 11).

Physiological Response

Experiments to determine the blocking action to morphine have been performed in rats, mice, dogs and monkeys by injecting suspensions of a 35% naltrexone-PLA composite in particle form in 7% CM-cellulose 7LF gel. The dosages used and the duration of the blocking action are summarized in Table I.

The duration of morphine antagonist activity in Sprague-Dawley rats and mice was determined by using the tail pinch test. Significant blocking action was observed throughout the 24-day test period for rats and 21 days for mice. No gross signs of tissue irritation

TABLE I

BLOCKING ACTION OF NALTREXONE-
PLA COMPOSITES

Animal	No. of Animals	Dose mg/kg	Blocking action Duration, day
Rats [20]	70	240	24
Dogs [22]	5	17	21-29
Monkeys [20]	4	30	20
Mice [21]	10	39	21

were found, but hair was lost in the implant area in the test with rats [20, 21].

The physiological response in dogs was determined by measuring the flexor reflex, the skin twitch reflex, the pulse rate and the pupillary diameter. The results showed a highly significant level of blockage of the effects of morphine for all parameters, except lowering of pulse rate, through the 21st day, and a significant level of blockage for the flexor reflex through the 29th day. Some irritant properties were observed and one dog out of six developed an abscess [22].

Antagonist activity was determined in Macaca mulatta monkeys by measuring the changes in morphine-induced prolongation of interblink time. Complete antagonism to the depressant effects of morphine on the blinking rate occurred 24 hours after antagonist injection. The estimated duration of statistically significant activity was approximately 20 days [20].

ANTICANCER AGENT COMPOSITES

The release rates of cytoxan and cis-dichlorodiammine-platinum (II) from PLA composites were determined. As shown by the amounts of N and P present in the cytoxan composites before and after the in vivo tests, an average of 67% of the administered dose was released over a 34-day test period. This result demonstrates the feasibility of a sustained delivery of drug from PLA composites. This feasibility was further substantiated by electron spectroscopy chemical analysis (ESCA) spectra of the composite recorded before implantation and at the end of the test (Fig. 12). The peaks of Cl and P atoms showed a considerable decrease in intensity at the end of the test.

Determination of the release rate of cytoxan by measuring the amounts of N and P excreted in urine was not performed since N and P compounds are normally present in urine.

The release rate of cis-dichlorodiammineplatinum (II), from PLA composites, determined from the amount of Pt in urine, was slow and decreased to a small amount after 18 days from implantation (Table II).

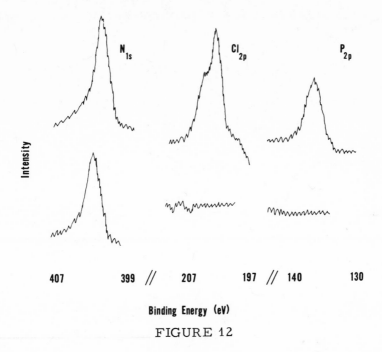

Binding Energy (eV)

FIGURE 12

TABLE II

AMOUNTS OF Pt AND CUMULATIVE PERCENT
OF DOSE EXCRETED IN URINE

Period Days	mg Pt in 4 days	Cum mg Pt	Cum % of dose
0- 4	0.88	0.88	1.87
4- 8	0.52	1.40	2.97
8-12	0.24	1.65	3.21
12-18	0.06	1.71	3.63
18-26	0.05	1.76	3.74
26-34	0.05	1.81	3.85

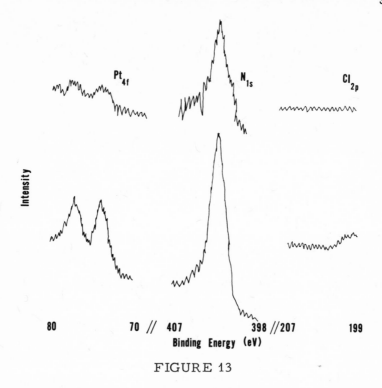

FIGURE 13

The cumulative amount of drug in the urine, expressed as percent of the administered dose, was 3.85, whereas the amount of drug released from the composite during the test, calculated from the amount of drug remaining in the film at the end of the test, was 9.3%. These results indicate that a significant amount of drug unaccounted for either remains sequestered within the animal or is eliminated through ways other than in the urine. The presence of large amounts of drug left in the composite at the end of the experiment is also shown by the ESCA spectra (Fig. 13). The relatively low amount of Pt compound in the surface of the original film, as shown by the electron energy spectra, is attributed to its very low solubility in the polymer and its low rate of diffusion. On the other hand, cytoxan being more soluble in the polymer appeared to a considerable extent in the surface of the original film. These solubility observations are further borne out by the physical appearance of the respective films, that of cytoxan being translucent and that of Pt compound opaque. At present, we are in the process of further studying the electron spectroscopic technique for measuring the diffusion rate of drugs in polymer films.

In addition, differences in the release of these two drugs can be attributed to differences in solubilities in water. The solubility of cytoxan in water is 40 g/1 [23] and that of cis-dichlorodiammine-platinum (II) is 2.2 g/1 [24].

These results prove the feasibility of a controlled release system for delivering anticancer agents and suggest that this concept of controlled release is of great potential for use in cancer therapy.

ACKNOWLEDGEMENTS

Supported by National Institute of Mental Health, Contract No. HSM 42-72-97.

The author gratefully acknowledges the assistance of Dr. Mario Sartori and Thomas D. Leafe of the University of Delaware, and Dr. Francis J. Meyer of Extracorporeal Medical Specialties, Inc., King of Prussia, Pa., 19406.

REFERENCES

1. Saunder, F. J. and Raymond, A. L., U. S. Patent 2,413,419 (1946).

2. Doyle, L. L. and Clewe, T. H., Amer. J. Obstet. Gynecol., 101, 564 (1968).

3. Mishell, D. R., Jr. and Lumkin, M. E., Fertil. Steril., 21, 99 (1970).

4. Roseman, T. J. and Higuchi, W. I., J. Pharm. Sci., 59, 353 (1970).

5. Roseman, T. J., ibid., 61, 46 (1972).

6. Woodland, J.H.R., Yolles, S., Blake, D. A., Helrich, M., and Meyer, F. J., J. Med. Chem., 16, 897 (1973).

7. Lazarus, J., Pagliery, M., and Lachman, L., J. Pharm. Sci., 53, 798 (1964).

8.   Farhadieh, B., Borodkin, S., and Buddenhagen, J. D.,
     ibid., 60, 209 (1971).

9.   Higuchi, T., ibid., 52, 1145 (1963).

10. Yolles, S., Eldridge, J. E., and Woodland, J.H.R., Polym.
     News, 1, 9 (1971).

11. Archer, S., in Narcotic Antagonists, M. C. Braude, et al.,
     Eds., Adv. Biochem. Psychopharmacol., 8, 549 (1974).

12. Newsweek, January 4, 1971.

13. Martin, W. R. and Sandquist, V. L., presented at the 34th
     Annual Meeting on Problems of Drug Dependence, Ann Arbor,
     Michigan, May 22-24, 1972.

14. Yolles, S., Leafe, T. D., Woodland, J.H.R., and Meyer,
     F. J., J. Pharm. Sci., (in press).

15. Yolles, S., Leafe, T. D., and Meyer, F. J., ibid., (in press).

16. Wall Street Journal, December 7, 1970.

17. Chem. Eng. News, February 19, 1973, p. 33.

18. Tanquary, A. C., Cowsar, D. R., and Lacey, R. E., Bull.
     So. Res. Inst., 25, 2 (1972).

19. Leafe, T. D., Sarner, S., Woodland, J.H.R., Yolles, S.,
     Blake, D. A., and Meyer, F. J., in Narcotic Antagonists,
     M. C. Braude, et al., Eds., Adv. Biochem.
     Psychopharmacol., 8, 569 (1974).

20. McCarthy, A., personal communication.

21. Reuning, R. H., personal communication.

22. Martin, W. R. and Sandquist, V. L., Arch. Gen. Psychiatry,
     30, 31 (1974).

23.   The Merck Index, 8th ed, Merck and Co., Inc., Rahway,
      New Jersey, 1968.

24.   Cleare, M. J. and Hoeschele, J. D., Bioinorg. Chem., 2,
      187 (1973).

POLYMERS IN BIOMEDICAL DEVICES: MATERIALS FOR ARTIFICIAL HEART AND CIRCULATORY ASSIST DEVICES

William S. Pierce

Department of Surgery, The Milton S. Hershey Medical Center of the Pennsylvania State University, Hershey, Pa.

Using currently available techniques, the cardiovascular surgeon is capable of correcting a wide variety of congenital heart defects, replacing damaged cardiac valves and blood vessels, and restoring blood flow to ischemic heart muscle. The next major frontier to be crossed concerns the replacement or substitution of damaged heart muscle, most commonly required in the patient who has sustained a major myocardial infarction. It is now recognized that if 30-40% of the left ventricular muscle is damaged, the cardiac chamber will be unable to generate power sufficient for patient survival in spite of the best forms of drug therapy currently available [1]. In some of these patients, there is reason to believe that temporary, i.e. weeks, mechanical cardiac assistance, possibly in the form of left atrial or left ventricle to aortic pumping, may be associated with improvement in existing left ventricular function, permitting the cardiac assist to be discontinued [2]. In patients with more severe forms of left ventricular failure, cardiac transplantation or heart replacement with a prosthetic device would appear to offer the only hope for patient survival.

For a variety of reasons, cardiac transplantation has advanced at a much more rapid pace than the development of the artificial heart [3]. However, formidable problems that exist regarding availability of donor hearts, as well as other factors, have led several groups, including our own, to develop implantable artificial hearts [4, 5, 6, 7].

Two of the major reasons why development of mechanical cardiac assist devices and artificial hearts has been so slow are unavailability of proper materials and a failure to appreciate certain design principles required for implantable blood handling devices.   Some investigators continue to believe that progress with the artificial heart must await development of new materials with "magic" properties including antithrombogenicity and superior mechanical characteristics.   It is our belief that adequate materials and know-how are presently available for the completion of this task, although improved materials may well facilitate the task.

GENERAL DESIGN FEATURES OF BLOOD PUMPS

At first thought, one might consider that the design principles employed in the heart-lung machine, used so commonly during cardiac operations, would serve as a basis for the design of implantable blood pumps.   Virtually all heart-lung machines employ valveless, roller-type pumps.   They are rather large in size, require relatively large amounts of power for operation, and provide continuous, rather than pulsatile, flow.   Continuous anticoagulation

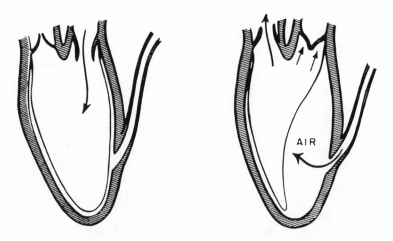

FIGURE 1.   General design of a blood pump suitable for implantation.   The pump features a flexible chamber whose opposite walls do not contact and some form of internal inlet and outlet valve. The pump is powered by fluid pulses introduced into the space between the rigid shell and flexible chamber.

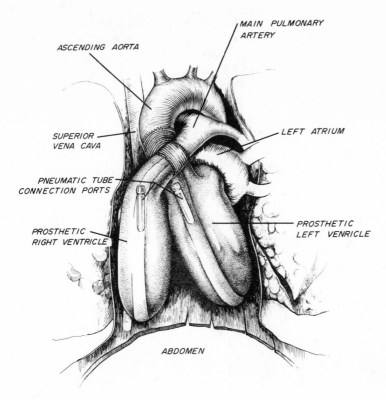

FIGURE 2. General design of the most successfully employed artificial hearts. The two pumps are positioned in the pericardial sac and are powered by air pulses from an external power source.

is employed and the tubing life is measured in hours rather than weeks or months. In contrast, successfully employed implanted blood pumps are of the sac, diaphragm, or concentric tube type. They employ inlet and outlet valves, are fluid powered, provide pulsatile flow, and their functional life is measured in months. Ideally, they can be used without complete anticoagulation. Figure 1 shows the general design of a blood pump suitable for use as an assist pump or for one ventricle of an artificial heart. Figure 2 shows the general design of an implanted, air-powered artificial heart.

While it is recognized by the author that implanted blood pumps will ultimately be driven directly by electromechanical conversion or by hydraulic power, it is apparent that all successes in this field to date have been with blood pumps powered by external pneumatic

units. Many problems remain to be solved before the pneumatic
blood pumps can be replaced by those capable of being powered by
the more compact, portable power sources. Only minor changes
will be required in the blood pump design.

POLYMERS SUITABLE FOR FABRICATION OF CIRCULA-
TORY ASSIST DEVICES AND THE ARTIFICIAL HEART

The use of materials for fabrication of prosthetic blood pumps
should be based, where possible, on materials already having a
good history when implanted in the cardiovascular system. Although experiences with polymers used within the cardiovascular
system are somewhat limited, valuable information is available
[8].

The most successful use of polymers in the cardiovascular
system is in the form of fabric grafts employed for replacement
of arteries 8 mm in diameter or larger. Both Teflon and Dacron
fabrics are widely employed, and have held up well for implantation periods of 15 years or more. Porous fabrics of this type
have little use in the pumping chamber of implanted blood pumps
where fluid under pressure is employed to power the devices and
the risk of fluid embolism is present.

Various rigid polymers have been implanted in the cardiovascular system, most frequently as components of prosthetic
cardiac valves. These materials have, in general, a shorter
history than the porous fabrics. Suitable materials for valve components include ultra-high density polyethylene and polypropylene.
Teflon has been satisfactorily used but is quite soft for most practical applications. While Delrin has been used for valve poppets,
it adsorbs a moderate amount of water, leading to a size increase.
Pyrolytic carbon, recently developed by Gulf-General Atomic, has
a smooth, hard, glass-like surface and is being used in a variety
of different prosthetic heart valves.

Rigid polymers have a variety of applications in the fabrication
of implantable blood pumps as housings, as blood-contacting components useful in valves, and as connectors to couple biologic tissue to the blood pump. Various rigid polymers which can be used
for fabrication of artificial heart components are available, although each has certain disadvantages (Table I).

TABLE I

PROBLEMS ASSOCIATED WITH RIGID POLYMERS USED IN
THE FABRICATION OF CARDIOVASCULAR PROSTHESES

Rigid polymer	Problem
Teflon	Very soft
Ultra high density poly-ethylene	Difficult to machine and polish
Polypropylene	Requires molding techniques
Delrin	Hygroscopic
Polycarbonate	Multiple inclusions (carbon)
Kel-F	Multiple inclusions Extremely expensive
Pyrolytic carbon	Fabrication difficult Brittle

The choice of a suitable elastomer is much more limited than
that of a rigid polymer. However, the selection of a proper elastomer is an absolute necessity for the fabrication of an implantable blood pump having a long-functioning life. Until several years
ago, silicone rubber served as the only suitable inert elastomer
for use in the vascular system. The poppet in the most widely
employed ball valve is fabricated of Silastic silicone rubber. Large
numbers of successful valve implants, using these poppets, have
been performed since 1961. A small percentage of these balls
have developed "ball variance" in which a lipid material has been
absorbed by the rubber, causing serious derangement in ball size
and mechanical properties [9]. A revised cure schedule, employed since 1967, has eliminated this problem. The major problem with the use of silicone rubber for blood pump fabrication centers around relatively poor mechanical properties, particularly

apparent when fabricated in the forms required for pump bladders. It must be pointed out that silicone rubber has nevertheless been employed successfully, i.e. without mechanical failure, provided that the design of the device is within the limits of the mechanical properties of the silicone rubber [7]. However, these design constraints may, in themselves, lead to thrombogenic pumps.

In 1961, Kolff and his group reported the fabrication of a variety of implantable cardiovascular devices using a polyurethane derived from a solution of Estane VC in tetrahydrofuran [10]. The material had acceptable biologic reactivity. Other groups, including our own, began using devices fabricated of Estane VC. A short time later, Mirkovitch and Kolff implanted a variety of polymers in muscle tissue of animals to learn how implantation affected the mechanical properties [11]. After one year of implantation, the polyurethane had been completely broken down. Polyurethanes were assumed to be a homogeneous group and were subsequently considered by many as unsuitable for biological use. Furthermore, most of the polyurethanes are not sufficiently elastic for

TABLE II

COMPARISON OF PROPERTIES OF SEGMENTED POLYURETHANE AND SILICONE RUBBER

Property	Segmented polyurethane*	Silicone rubber**
Tensile strength (lb/sq in)	6700	1290
Stress at 100% elongation (lb/sq in)	850	160
Elongation at break (%)	750	560
Hardness (Shore A)	75	50
Specific gravity	1.1	1.1

*Polymer T-125, E. I. du Pont de Nemours and Co., Inc.
**Silastic 9711, Dow Corning Corp., Midland, Michigan

fabrication of useful prostheses. In 1966, a materials program
was launched at the National Institutes of Health to locate a material suitable for fabrication of thin-walled tubing for use in an implantable roller-type assist pump. After approximately a dozen
materials had been discarded on the basis of mechanical properties
or difficulty in fabrication, a Lycra thread was obtained. Tubes
were subsequently fabricated from a segmented polyurethane solution having the same chemical structure as the Lycra fiber [12]*.
The mechanical properties were outstanding (Table II) and the polyether linkage in the polymer insured that hydrolysis would not
occur. Lee-White clotting time determinations were performed in
test tubes fabricated of segmented polyurethane and showed clotting
times to be equal to, or longer than, those obtained in silicone
rubber tubes. Vena caval rings fabricated of segmented polyurethane had a behavior similar to silicone rubber rings with regard
to thrombus formation. The mechanical properties of segmented
polyurethane appear relatively unchanged following in vivo use for
roller pump tubing or for pump bladders (Table III).

Two other elastomers also appear to be suitable for fabrication of prosthetic blood pumps. One is a type of segmented polyurethane produced by the Stanford Research Institute [13]. The
chemical structure of this material is similar to that of Biomer
although the mechanical properties are apparently inferior.

A different group of elastomers, Avcothanes, represent a
family of copolymers of polyurethane and silicone rubber [14].
This material is suitable for intravascular use and has been widely
employed in the fabrication of intraaortic balloons. The fabrication techniques are more difficult than those for Biomer.

THE BLOOD-MATERIAL INTERFACE

Perhaps the most important controversy in the area of implantable blood pump development today concerns the blood-contacting surface or pump lining. At the present time, it is not
clear if the pump lining should be fabricated with an extremely
smooth blood-contacting surface, with a fabric surface on which
a fibrin membrane will form, or with a fabric surface which has
been seeded with cells (Table IV).

---

*Currently available as Biomer, Ethicon, Inc., Somerville, N. J.

TABLE III

MECHANICAL PROPERTIES OF SEGMENTED POLYURETHANE BEFORE
AND AFTER USE IN A CIRCULATORY ASSIST PUMP

Property	Roller pump* Continuous assist in calf 6 days 250 rpm		Sac pump** Continuous assist in calf 11 weeks 120 bpm	
	Control	Test specimen	Control	Test specimen
Tensile strength (psi)	6650	6450	3108	3039
Stress at 100% elonga- tion (psi)	857	852	596	631
Elongation at break (%)	755	738	518	498

*Polymer T-125, E. I. du Pont de Nemours and Co., Inc.
**Biomer, Ethicon, Inc.

Roller pump and sac pump samples were of different size

TABLE IV

THREE SURFACES UNDER INVESTIGATION FOR
FABRICATION OF IMPLANTABLE BLOOD PUMPS

A. Nonthrombogenic Smooth Surface
   1. Hydrodynamic method (proper de-
       sign, material, smoothness)
   2. Heparin bonding (GBH, TDMAC)

B. Fibrin Membrane Surface
   1. Dacron fibrils
   2. Velour fabric
   3. Knit fabric

C. Cell-Seeded Surface
   1. Bovine fetal fibroblasts

The smooth surface concept is based on the fact that the lining of the heart and blood vessels is smooth. The precise definition of smooth is not presently known, but certainly defects must be smaller than the diameter of a blood platelet (3 microns), the smallest of the blood elements and the most important in initiating thrombus formation. Perhaps more important is the chemical composition of the smooth polymer. Plasma proteins adsorb in different concentrations to different polymer surfaces and appear to influence platelet adhesion [15]. Considerable work has been done to develop smooth surfaces to which heparin can be bonded, thus rendering the surface antithrombogenic. Of the bonding techniques, the graphite-benzalkonium-heparin, and TDMAC-heparin surfaces have been the most useful, but loss of bonded heparin over a relatively short period, i.e. days, has led to a further search [16, 17]. The smooth surface concept has been successfully employed in the form of poppets and discs for ball and disc-type cardiac valves, struts for a variety of valve cages, and for arterial replacement when special effort has been taken to eliminate anastomotic problems [18, 19]. On the other hand, most of the implantable blood pumps with smooth linings employed to date have imperfect surfaces as a result of fabrication techniques or inclusion of foreign substances. Nonadherent thrombi form in the sac and subsequently embolize.

The fabric surface concept is based on a long, generally successful experience with arterial replacement by knitted or woven
fabric-type tubular grafts. In most instances, such grafts develop
a glistening intimal lining by extension of the intima from the arterial anastomoses and by direct fibroblastic invasion of the interstices of the graft. The exciting idea to employ a nonporous fabric
covering to blood-contacting surfaces of a blood pump was developed by Liotta and Hall [20]. The concept was rather thoroughly
studied in a left ventricular assist in calves and subsequently employed clinically in a similar device [21]. The idea has been employed by several other groups in both assist pumps and the artificial heart [4, 22]. Velour, woven, and flocked surfaces have
been studied. The surface which develops is considerably different from that seen in the arterial grafts because the pump surface
is nonporous and all nutrition to the lining must occur from the
blood-contacting surface. The autologous lining that develops consists of fibrin plus cellular islands containing fibroblasts and collagen. In areas of poor washout of the pump, a lining 1 cm or
more in thickness may form. Since nutrients cannot reach the
deepest parts of this lining, necrosis and dislodgement of the partially organized fibrin surface may occur [23].

Bernhard and his group have extended the concept of the fabric
surface by actually seeding the pump bladder with bovine fetal
fibroblasts grown in tissue culture [24]. The cells are incubated
in the flock lined pump bladder for approximately one hour prior
to pump implantation. This technique appears to facilitate organization of the pump lining. The blood-contacting surfaces of the
pumps, examined 1-2 months postimplantation, showed broad sheets
of fibroblasts and collagen firmly fixed to the stationary flexing
surfaces of the pump [22]. These studies have now been extended
to nine months [25].

It is important to recognize that the precise chemical structure and surface finish of the polymer are of primary importance
in preventing thrombus formation in the smooth surface concept
(Table I), whereas the structural polymers employed in the fibrin
membrane surface or cell-seeded surface serve only to insure
adequate mechanical strength. Thrombus prevention is based entirely on the biological surface coating.

TABLE V

FACTORS INFLUENCING THROMBOEMBOLUS FORMATION IN PROSTHETIC BLOOD PUMPS

1. Pump design

2. Blood-material interface

3. Flow rate

4. Modification of coagulation mechanism

EXPERIENCE WITH THE USE OF DIFFERENT ELASTOMERS IN CIRCULATORY ASSIST DEVICES AND THE ARTIFICIAL HEART

It is difficult to make statements at the present time as to which materials or surfaces are optimal for fabrication of blood pumps. Evaluation of mechanical properties can naturally be accomplished by bench testing. In unlined pumps, the fabrication materials are important in preventing thromboemboli, the major factor currently limiting clinical use of these devices. However, thrombus formation is also dependent on other factors (Table V). All four are operant in every experiment. Failure to properly account for any one factor may lead to thrombus formation.

The five major elastomer-lining combinations that have been employed for prosthetic blood pumps over the past 15 years are listed in Table VI. The earliest pumps were fabricated of silicone rubber with no special lining. Pump design and proper fit represented major problems. Failure in one-third of the devices was a result of disruption of the silicone rubber bladder. Increased survival of animals was achieved when a fabric surface was employed as a lining but, as mentioned earlier, progressive fibrin buildup represented a serious drawback of this method. However, pumps fabricated using the flock technique on silicone rubber bladders have permitted Kolff's group to extend survival in calves with implanted artificial hearts from 100 hours to a month or more, a quantum jump in this field [4]. An improvement in pump life

TABLE VI

ELASTOMERS AND LININGS EMPLOYED FOR
PROSTHETIC BLOOD PUMP FABRICATION

Material	Major investigator	Problems	Usefulness (+4 = ideal)
Silicone rubber	Akutsu, DeBakey, Kolff, Nosé	Mechanical failure Thromboembolism	+1
Silicone rubber with fabric or flock surface	DeBakey, Kolff	Fibrin buildup Thromboembolism Embolization of flocking	+2
Polyurethane with flocking	Bernhard	As above	+2
Polyurethane with cell-seeded surface	Bernhard	Difficulty in preparation Progressive tissue buildup	+3
Segmented polyurethane	Kolff, Pierce	Thromboembolism	+3

occurred with the use of polyurethane as a base elastomer for flocking but progressive tissue buildup plus embolization of Dacron fibrils imposed serious limitations.

A major advance occurred in 1969 when Bernhard and the group at the Boston Children's Hospital seeded the flocked surface with bovine fetal fibroblast cells, incubated the bladder for 60 minutes, and then implanted the pumps [22]. Calves have undergone long-term left ventricular-aortic assist pumping for nine months with this system. This surface is more highly organized than the flocked, unseeded surface, and is composed of fibroblasts

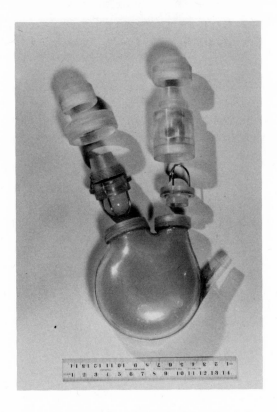

FIGURE 3. An exploded view of the left ventricle-aortic assist pump. The segmented polyurethane sac is housed within a rigid polycarbonate shell. Ball type inlet and outlet valves are housed within polycarbonate connectors.

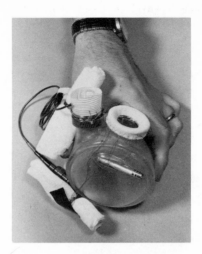

FIGURE 4A. The prosthetic left ventricle is a segmented polyurethane sac housed in an epoxy shell. A Dacron fabric sewing
ring with preplaced atrial sutures serves as the inlet connection
while a Dacron graft is anastomosed to the aorta. An implanted
arterial pressure transducer is fixed in the Dacron graft to moni-
tor aortic pressure.

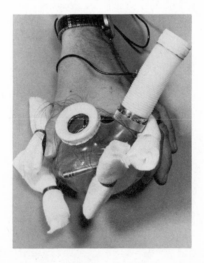

FIGURE 4B. The right ventricular counterpart of the artificial
heart. A similar inlet connector is employed. A quick-connect
is used to anastomose the Dacron graft to the pulmonary artery.
Again, an implantable pressure transducer is employed to moni-
tor pulmonary artery pressure.

and fibrocytes with strands of collagen. Major problems with the
seeded flocked surface are listed below and further work is required to resolve these important concerns:

     1. Difficulty in preparation
     2. Time required for preparation (emergency
         use of pump)
     3. Stability of surface
     4. Antigenicity
     5. Progressive tissue buildup
     6. Adhesion of surface to polyurethane
     7. Species variation in cellular growth

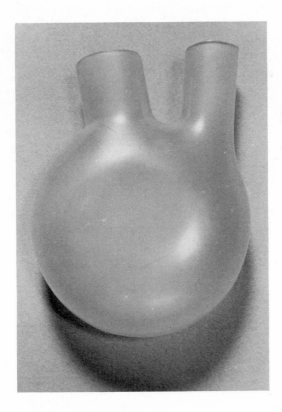

FIGURE 5. The sac design employed in the left ventricular
assist pump and in the artificial heart. The form must be crushed
for removal from the inside of the sac.

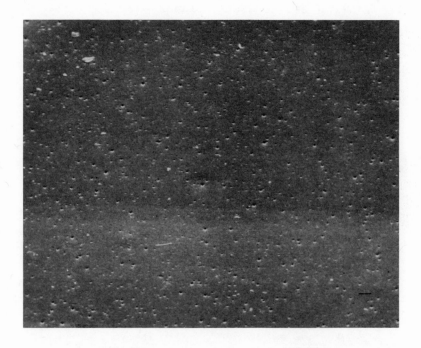

FIGURE 6. Scanning electron micrograph of the blood-contacting surface of a segmented polyurethane sac fabricated over a silicone rubber dispersion coated form.   A. Original magnification x500.

B. Original magnification x1000. The appropriate size of a red
blood cell is indicated by the length of the bar in each photograph.

FIGURE 7. Scanning electron micrograph of the inner surface of
segmented polyurethane film cast on a warm glass slide.
A. Original magnification x1000; the vertical line represents a
scratch made in the surface to permit precise focusing.

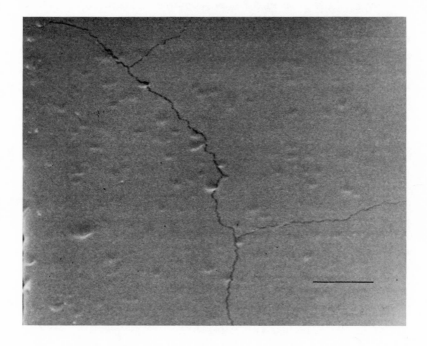

B. Original magnification x2500. The lines represent fractures
in the gold-palladium coating on the polymer. The approximate
size of a red blood cell is indicated by the length of the bar in each
photograph. Note the improved surface when compared with
Figure 6.

CURRENT EXPERIENCE WITH THE UNLINED SEG-
MENTED POLYURETHANE SAC IN A CIRCULA-
TORY ASSIST DEVICE AND ARTIFICIAL HEART

In 1971, our group directed its efforts to further evaluation
of the smooth, unlined, blood-contacting surface. A sac-type
pump was designed which could be used as an assist device for
left ventricular to aortic pumping (Fig. 3) . With minor modifications, two such pumps could be employed for total heart replacement (Fig. 4) . The sac was seam-free, segmented polyurethane
with special attention directed toward obtaining the smoothest
possible defect-free surface.

The fabrication of smooth, seam-free sacs of segmented polyurethane has been a difficult but important task. The sac design
requires that the sac form be crushable for removal after application of the final dip coating of segmented polyurethane (Fig. 5).
The polyurethane solvent employed, N, N-dimethylacetamide,
attacks the surface of many potentially useful form materials.
Metals, waxes, silicone rubber, and glass appear to be the usable
form materials. The forms we have most recently used are fabricated of hollow polyethylene wax. The frequent occurrence of one
or more small defects and a flash line has made the form rejection
rate excessive. The wax form is now coated with a silicone rubber dispersion. Scanning electron micrographs have revealed
multiple surface defects in polyurethane cast on this surface, consisting of bubbles and craters, approximately 1/4-1 micron in
diameter (Fig. 6). We have recently fabricated segmented polyurethane over warmed glass slides with considerable improvement in the scanning electron micrographic appearance of the cast
polyurethane surface (Fig. 7). Fabrication of the sacs over glass
forms in a dust-free environment is presently being considered.

Pumps employing segmented polyurethane sacs fabricated
over silicone rubber dispersions have been used for left ventricular assists in ten calves [26]. The average period of continuous
assist was six weeks while the longest period was over eight months
(Fig. 8). No mechanical pump failures occurred. In the last three
animals assisted, there was continuous high blood flow, an improved blood-contacting surface, and continuous use of some form
of coagulation modification (generally Coumadin). Thromboembolic
phenomena did not occur in these animals. Encouraged by these
results, a small number of similarly designed pumps have been
employed for total heart replacement in the calf. The last calf

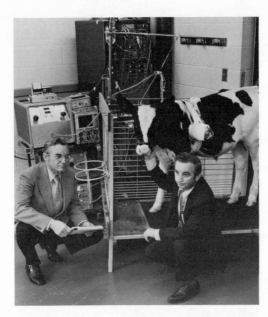

FIGURE 8.   Long-term left ventricular-aortic pumping in the calf.
The pump shown in Figure 3 was placed in the paracorporeal location.   One such calf has undergone over eight months of continuous
circulatory assistance.

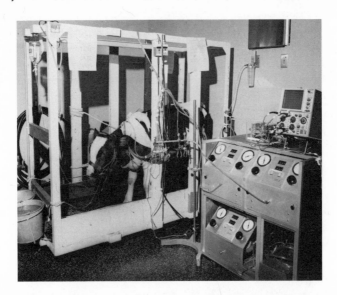

FIGURE 9.   Total heart replacement with the pumps shown in
Figure 4.   The calf ate well and remained standing for long periods
of time.   He died suddenly, 12 days after operation, when a strut
on the inlet valve broke.

survived for 12 days, the cause of death being breakage of a strut on a Bjork-Shiley valve (Fig. 9). Several strands of white thrombus were found in the pumps and renal emboli were present.

SUMMARY AND CONCLUSIONS

Considerable work has been performed over a 16-year period to develop mechanical circulatory assist devices and an artificial heart. At the present time, the general problems of mechanical design and device fit have been solved. Mechanical failures should rarely occur during animal experimentation.

The major problem encountered with left ventricular assist devices and the artificial heart in 1974 is thromboembolism. Resolution of this problem is largely based on a suitable blood-material interface. Two interfaces show particular promise at the present time. In one system, a flocked polyurethane bladder is seeded with bovine fetal fibroblasts prior to pump implantation, resulting in the formation of a nonthrombogenic surface of fibroblasts and collagen.

We have followed an alternate and somewhat simpler approach in which an extremely smooth, segmented polyurethane, blood-contacting surface is employed. The results of our initial series of calf experiments have been encouraging. We believe that the use of pump sacs fabricated of extremely smooth, seam-free segmented polyurethane, in conjunction with agents which modify the coagulation mechanism, will provide an important step toward attaining the goal of safe, long-term blood pumping with a mechanical circulatory assist device or the artificial heart.

ACKNOWLEDGEMENTS

Supported in part by U. S. Public Health Service grant 5 RO1 HL13426; Contract NO1-HV-3-2966, Division of Heart and Vascular Diseases, NHLI; and the Jane B. Barsumian Trust Fund.

The work presented represents the results of The Pennsylvania State University Artificial Heart group. The author would like to express special thanks to Mr. Mark Kurusz for preparing the scanning photomicrographs and to Mrs. Catharine Knox for her excellent assistance.

REFERENCES

1. Page, D., Caulfield, J., Kastor, J., DeSantis, R., and
    Saunders, G., New Engl. J. Med., 235, 133 (1971).

2. Buckley, M. J., Craver, J. M., Gold, H. K., Mundth,
    E. D., Daggett, W. M., and Austen, W. G., Circulation,
    48 (Suppl. 3), 90 (1973).

3. Stinson, E., Griepp, R., Bieber, C., and Shumway, N.,
    J. Thorac. Cardiov. Surg., 63, 344 (1972).

4. Kawai, J., Volder, J., Donovan, F., and Kolff, W., Ann.
    Surg., 179, 362 (1974).

5. Kito, Y., Takagi, H., Honda, T., Gibson, W., and Akutsu,
    T., Trans. Amer. Soc. Artif. Intern. Organs, 19, 573
    (1973).

6. Nosé, Y., Tajima, K., Imai, Y., Klain, M., Mrava, G.,
    Schriber, K., Urbanek, K., and Ogawa, H., ibid., 17,
    482 (1971).

7. Ross, J., Akers, W., O'Bannon, W., Spargo, W., Serrato,
    M., Fuqua, J., Ruark, B., Wieting, D., Kennedy, J., and
    DeBakey, M., ibid., 18, 168 (1972).

8. Boretos, J. W., Concise Guide to Biomedical Polymers,
    Charles C. Thomas, Springfield, Ill., 1973.

9. Stan, A., Pierie, W., Raible, D., Edwards, M., Siposs,
    G., and Hancock, W., Circulation, 34 (Suppl. 1), 115
    (1966).

10. Dreyer, B., Akutsu, T., and Kolff, W., J. Appl. Physiol.,
    15, 18 (1960).

11. Mirkovitch, V., Akutsu, T., and Kolff, W., Trans. Amer.
    Soc. Artif. Intern. Organs, 8, 79 (1962).

12. Boretos, J. W. and Pierce, W. S., Science, 158, 1481
    (1967).

13. Lyman, D., Brash, J., and Klein, K., in Proceedings of the Artificial Heart Program Conference, R. J. Hegyeli, Ed., National Heart Institute Artificial Heart Program, Washington, D.C., 1969, p. 113.

14. Nyilas, E., Proc. Ann. Conf. Eng. Med. Biol., 12, 147 (1970).

15. Kim, S., Lee, R., Oster, H., Lentz, D., Coleman, L., Andrade, J., and Olsen, D., Trans. Amer. Soc. Artif. Intern. Organs, 20, 449 (1974).

16. Gott, V., Whiffen, J., and Dutton, R., Science, 142, 1293 (1963).

17. Grode, G., Crowley, J., and Falb, R., J. Biomed. Mater. Res., 6, Symp. No. 3, 77 (1972).

18. Starr, A., and Edwards, M., Ann. Surg., 154, 726 (1961).

19. Sparks, C., Ann. Thorac. Surg., 2, 585 (1966).

20. Liotta, D., Hall, C. W., Akers, W. W., Villanueva, A., O'Neal, R., and DeBakey, M., Trans. Amer. Soc. Artif. Intern. Organs, 12, 129 (1966).

21. DeBakey, M. E., Amer. J. Cardiol., 27, 3 (1971).

22. Bernhard, W., Husain, M., Robinson, T., Button, L., Frieze, S., and Curtis, G., J. Thorac. Cardiov. Surg., 58, 801 (1969).

23. Sharp, W., Taylor, B., Wright, J., Nuwayser, E., Miller, B., Hampton, G., and Wilson, C., Trans. Amer. Soc. Artif. Intern. Organs, 18, 232 (1972).

24. Bernhard, W., Husain, M., George, J., and Curtis, G., Surgery, 66, 284 (1969).

25. Personal communication.

26. Pierce, W., Brighton, J., O'Bannon, W., Donachy, J., Phillips, W., Landis, D., White, W., and Waldhausen, J., Ann. Surg. (in press).

IMPROVED BIOMATERIALS FOR ARTIFICIAL
LUNG MEMBRANES

Warren M. Zapol and John Ketteringham

Artificial Lung Laboratory, Department of Anesthesia, Harvard Medical School at the Massachusetts General Hospital, and Arthur D. Little, Inc., Cambridge, Massachusetts

The membrane lung is a prosthetic device presently used in an extracorporeal blood circuit to partially exchange respiratory gases when the function of the natural lung is severely compromised, or for total gas exchange during cardiac surgery. When used for respiratory insufficiency, the membrane lung avoids the complications of conventional ventilator therapy which arise from high airway pressures and inspired oxygen concentrations. By preventing both hypoxia and hypercapnea, the membrane lung can maintain life while otherwise fatal pulmonary damage receives therapy and heals [1, 2].

Membrane lungs transfer oxygen to the venous blood and remove carbon dioxide from it by transport through synthetic polymer membranes. This gentle process minimizes the progressive destruction of blood cells and denaturation of plasma proteins observed with contemporary disc and bubble blood oxygenators. With less blood damage, the use of membrane lungs in long-term (1-15 days) partial respiratory support is now a promising clinical therapy. Approximately twenty humans have survived perfusion for severe acute respiratory failure [3].

The development of a suitable membrane for an artificial lung poses different problems than that for the dramatically successful artificial kidney in which blood is contacted with a dialyzing fluid also across a synthetic hydrophilic membrane. While the body can tolerate periods of several days without renal function and therapeutic dialysis of urea and accumulated substances can take place intermittently for periods of several hours at blood flow rates of 200-400 ml per minute, tolerance to loss of lung function is only minutes; blood must be oxygenated and carbon dioxide removed continuously at blood flow rates of 3-6 liters per minute in order to sustain life. Contact with 3-6 square meters of hydrophobic membrane occurs in the membrane lung, therefore placing a premium on blood compatibility. In addition, in devices of manageable size, total gas transfer across the membrane lung must rival the natural lung (250 ml per minute of oxygen and carbon dioxide in a resting adult).

The basic requirements of materials for use in the membrane lung are:

1. They must have high oxygen and carbon dioxide permeability.

2. They should be chemically stable without leachable moieties and be blood compatible, minimizing thrombosis, platelet activation and injury, and protein denaturation.

3. They must be strong, pinhole-free and capable of withstanding a pressure gradient of 15 psi from the blood side without leaking.

4. They must be capable of sterilization preferably by ethylene oxide or by autoclaving.

5. They should be easily fabricated into pinhole-free membranes (containing a supporting component if necessary) with a surface conformation which can be designed to augment secondary blood flow against the surface.

6. The basic cost of the material and ease of fabrication must permit economical disposable devices to be constructed.

The major challenge of developing appropriate membrane materials is to combine adequate gas exchange properties with blood compatibility. These parameters are related because if gas permeability is low, larger membrane areas must be placed in con-

tact with the blood. Even when promising combinations of properties are found, difficulties of fabrication can lead to prohibitively
high costs. In addition, advances in the hemodynamic design of
blood oxygenators, particularly in the augmentation of secondary
flow to minimize stagnant blood layers adjacent to the membrane
surface, have placed increasing demands on the gas permeability
of the membranes [4, 5, 6]. Close attention to the purity and
smoothness of the membrane surfaces has been shown to reduce
platelet damage and heparin requirements to safer levels [7].
Recently, several advances have been made in membrane technology which suggest that inexpensive artificial lungs with high
gas transfer performance and minimal blood trauma can be anticipated.

GAS PERMEABILITY OF MEMBRANES

Few materials offer high enough gas permeability for use as
membranes in typical thicknesses of 50-125 microns. The first
membrane to be used in a practical artificial lung was Teflon,
chosen primarily because of its availability in thin sheets of large
area and its fair blood compatibility [8]. The gas permeability of
Teflon is very low and major blood leaks through these thin membranes (6-12 microns) were common.

Methods of preparing thin membranes of silica-filled silicone
rubber (SFSR) were developed during the early 1960s [9], although
difficulties with quality control, particularly with respect to pin-
holes and high cost, persist to the present. Silicone rubber has
the highest specific gas permeability of any polymer yet studied,
and pure filler-free silicone rubber (FFSR) has been shown to
minimize thrombosis as well as platelet sequestration [7]. The
chief drawbacks of the silicone rubbers are their low cohesive
strengths and difficulty of fabrication which requires 30-40 volume
percent of silica filler and at times casting upon supporting woven
or knit fabrics of Dacron, nylon, or glass monofilament to achieve
adequate mechanical properties.

Silicone rubber membranes are presently the common membranes in commercially available artificial lungs. Typical properties are:

Tensile strength	1, 250 lb/sq in
Specific gravity	1.2
Tear strength	9 lb
Elongation	350%
Thickness	50-300 μ
O_2 Permeability*	50 (16)
CO_2 Permeability*	270 (97)

Also available are copolymers of silicone rubber with polycarbon-ate (MEM 213 - General Electric Company; properties given above in parenthesis).

Burns and Melrose [10], and more recently Kolobow and Spragg [11], have extensively studied dispersion casting of sili-cone rubber, especially with regard to pinhole formation and weak areas which become holes under stress. Membrane defects were often traced to undispersed silica filler aggregates. Kolobow and Spragg found that major improvement in membrane quality was achieved by removing these aggregates from 20% silicone rubber stock in toluene by centrifugation at 10, 000 g for four hours. Careful measurement of the burst strength of the membrane re-vealed that 2-4% heat-activated 2, 4-dichlorobenzoyl peroxide catalyst yielded maximum strength. In addition, postcuring the membrane in a nitrogen atmosphere with ultraviolet irradiation increased tensile strength by 30%. Kolobow and Spragg were able to cast, on pure aluminum foil, excellent quality 50-75 μ thick fabric-reinforced silicone membranes. These membranes have now become standard in their spiral coil membrane lung.

While some of the basic disadvantages of silicone rubber mem-branes have been partly overcome, particularly with regard to fabrication, they remain costly and their blood compatibility is still too poor to allow perfusion without systemic anticoagulation (see later). There remains considerable incentive to find other polymers and membrane configurations to improve or equal the gas permeability of the thin rubbers, hopefully with enhanced blood compatibility.

---

*Units are $\dfrac{\text{cc gas (NTP) cm thick}}{\text{sec, sq cm, cm Hg}}$ x 10^{-9}

Two potentially successful approaches have recently been developed:

1. The complete coating of ultrathin membranes on porous substrates [12, 13], and

2. The use of microporous membrane materials [14].

Two main ultrathin membrane polymers have been developed and fabricated into ultrathin membranes, the polyalkylsulfones [15] and ethylcellulose perfluorobutyrate [16].

Polyalkylsulfones

The polyalkylsulfones (PAS) appear to promise an important and unique combination of five factors:

relatively high gas permeability

promising blood compatibility

opportunities for chemical and physical modification of properties

ease of fabrication, and

the promise of inexpensiveness

Polyalkylsulfones are copolymers of α-olefins and sulfur dioxide which were first reported as long ago as 1915 [17], and characterized as high molecular weight materials in 1934 [18]. The polymer series used in membrane fabrication was first prepared and characterized in 1971 by Crawford and Gray [19]. The general method of preparation is as follows:

A charge of excess liquid sulfur dioxide is introduced into a heavy walled container cooled in a dry ice-isopropanol bath. The greater proportion of the α-olefin is introduced and stirred to form a suspension of the excess liquid sulfur dioxide in the sulfur dioxide-olefin complex. The catalyst, t-butylhydroperoxide, is mixed in the remaining α-olefin and added with stirring to the reaction mixture. Rapid polymerization occurs at a temperature controlled between 25°C and 35°C. After several hours, the excess sulfur dioxide is vented.

$$CH_3(CH_2)_nCH = CH_2 + SO_2 \longrightarrow CH_3(CH_2)_n - CH - CH_2 \longrightarrow$$

$$\left[-CH - CH_2 - \overset{\overset{O}{\|}}{\underset{\underset{O}{\|}}{S}} - \right]_x$$
$$\underset{\underset{CH_3}{|}}{(CH_2)_n}$$

The product is first dissolved in chloroform and then precipitated by methanol. Purification may be continued by repeating
this solvent precipitation. The product is a white waxy solid with
a molecular weight between 120,000 and 4,000,000, depending on
reaction conditions. To achieve satisfactory physical and mechanical properties, no additional plasticizers or fillers are necessary.
Low crystallinity, absence of significant crosslinking, a mobile
polymer backbone, self-plasticization and sterically nonhindered
pendant groups maximize polymer gas permeability. In these respects, (PAS) is somewhat analogous to silicone rubber. Crawford
and Gray have postulated that the aliphatic side chains plasticize
the material up to C_{16}, but at C_{18} the side chains begin to crystallize, causing the observed increase in tensile strength and fall in
gas permeability. Uninhibited rotation about the carbon-carbon
and carbon-sulfur bonds of the backbone is probable: dipole interaction between the backbone sulfone groups will be inhibited by the
side chains, characteristics again compatible with high gas permeability.

The PAS materials prepared to date soften at about 75°C and
steam sterilization will not be possible, but preliminary results
indicate that ethylene oxide, radiation, and alcohol sterilization
are feasible. PAS is soluble in a wide range of organic solvents,
permitting solvent casting of pinhole-free thin unsupported membranes. More important, ultrathin membranes may be coated onto microporous substrates [13]. A successful technique developed
to fabricate these latter membranes has been to use, as substrate,
a material with an average pore size substantially smaller than the
molecules of the high molecular weight polymer. During coating

with PAS, the solvent penetrates the substrate but the polymer remains in a thin adherent layer on the surface. The resulting surface is remarkably smooth, and, as shown in Figure 1B, masks the surface roughness of the substrate (Fig. 1A).

Ethylcellulose Perfluorobutyrate

This recently synthesized polymer has been described by Rozelle and Petersen of the North Star Research Institute [16]. It is synthesized from ethyl cellulose by standard polymer chemistry procedures. The resulting resin is purified by solvent extraction and vacuum drying techniques. It has been further characterized by infrared spectroscopy, elemental analyses, and molecular weight determinations. A membrane float casting process has been developed: a solution of the fluoropolymer is placed in a hopper above a tank of water and allowed to flow through a slit orifice at the bottom of the hopper and down an inclined glass plate onto the water surface. There the solution spreads spontaneously over the water surface. A gelled polymer film is formed as the solvent migrates into the water. The film is drawn away from the point of gelation at a controlled rate by lamination to a moving belt of support material as the belt lifts the film from the water surface. A variation of this process was successfully used to produce ultrathin fluoropolymer membranes (bonded by a thin layer of silicone adhesive) to Tyvek, a spun bonded polyolefin support material. It may be used equally well with nonwoven polypropylene or polyester backing materials. Currently, solution casting of this polymer is being investigated.

Ethylcellulose perfluorobutyrate has excellent tensile strength (3,500 psi) and high rigidity, yet it is neither a brittle material nor a rubber-like material. Being a cellulosic material, its film-forming and handling characteristics are excellent. Therefore, the possibility of asymmetric membrane fabrication is being explored. Other properties of this fluoropolymer include oxygen and carbon dioxide permeability about 1/10th those of polydimethyl-siloxane, a critical surface energy of about 20 dynes/cm, 20,000 psi tensile modulus, 50-60% elongation at break, very good hydrolytic resistance at neutral pH, the ability to withstand steam and ethylene oxide sterilization, and excellent film-forming characteristics.

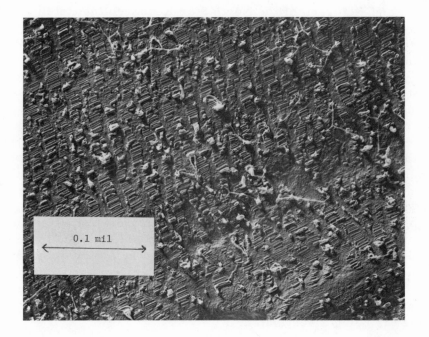

FIGURE 1. Scanning electron micrographs of ultrathin membrane surfaces. A. Uncoated microporous polypropylene (Celgard) - x16,000.

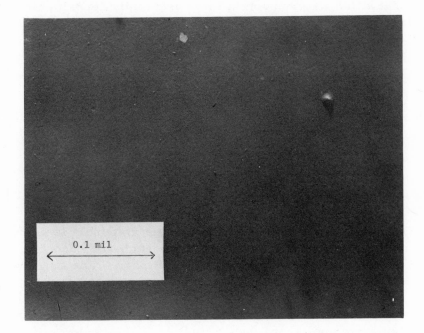

B. 0.1 mil thick PAS on microporous polypropylene (Celgard) - x16, 000.

Porous Membranes

Porous membrane materials have extremely high gas permeabilities. Membrane lungs have been constructed of porous polypropylene (Celgard; Celanese Corp.), porous Teflon (Gore-Tex; Gore Corp.), and porous silicone-cellulose (Rhône-Poulenc Corp.) [20]. Their blood compatibility is controversial: some argue that the intrinsic blood gas interface is inherently damaging to the blood citing rapid platelet destruction in human bypass; others argue that a thin watery protein layer is rapidly deposited to bridge the pores. Nevertheless, other problems of using porous materials in membrane lungs have been encountered [21]:

high water vapor transport

flooding of the pores (edema of
the prosthetic lung)

infection

gas embolization

While gas permeability of these porous materials is extremely high, the potentially very high rate of gas exchange cannot be realized due to blood film limitations even in membrane lungs with induced secondary flow.

Table I lists the specific permeabilities of the polymer materials mentioned and others under study.

The maximum permeation rates of gas through these materials obviously depends on their thickness and porosity: thin film and microporous membranes show considerably higher permeation rates than homogeneous membranes. Table II lists comparative figures for some typical membranes.

In conventional spiral coil, flat sheet (sandwich), or hollow fiber membrane lungs, when membranes of relatively high gas permeability are used at common blood flow rates, the oxygen transfer rate is limited by the blood film resistance and is independent of the membrane permeability [23]. On the other hand, the carbon dioxide permeation rate is limited by the membrane permeability and varies with the properties of the membrane.

TABLE I

GAS PERMEABILITY OF POLYMERS USED
IN MEMBRANE LUNGS [22]

Material	Permeability* O_2	Permeability* CO_2
Silicone rubber	50	270
Silicone rubber/poly-carbonate (MEM 213)	16	97
Polyalkylsulfone	6	25
Polyethylenecellulose per-fluorobutyrate	5	25
Teflon (as film)	1.1	2.5

$$* \quad \frac{cc, \ cm \ thick}{sq \ cm, \ sec, \ cm \ Hg} \times 10^{-9}$$

Measurements of gas-to-blood transport rates of oxygen and carbon dioxide were made in a special cell with reproducible blood channel dimensions and blood shear rate. While carbon dioxide permeabilities showed good correlation with gas-to-gas measurements, oxygen permeability was relatively similar for all membranes and depended only on the blood flow rate and surface texture which controls the blood boundary layer thickness through which the oxygen must diffuse.

Table III gives comparative data for several membranes under blood flow and gas partial pressure gradients found in conventional membrane lungs. In parenthesis, the maximum membrane oxygen permeability which would be achieved in the absence of the rate limiting blood film is given. This value has become important with the development of secondary flow augmented oxygenators [4, 5, 6] which disturb the boundary layer and require membranes of higher intrinsic oxygen permeability. The thin skinned PAS and polyfluorinated cellulose membrane appear especially suited for these devices.

TABLE II

COMPARATIVE MEMBRANE PERMEATION RATES OF
AVAILABLE MEMBRANE MATERIALS [22]

Material	Construction	Overall thickness μ	Membrane thickness μ	Permeation rate* O_2	Permeation rate* CO_2
Silicone rubber	Reinforced with Dacron knit	190	160	140	770
MEM-213	Homogeneous film	50	50	170	730
Ultrathin PAS	Coated porous poly-propylene	25	2.5	1100	4600
Ultrathin poly-fluorinated cellulose	Coated Tyvek	175	2.5	880	4700
Porous poly-propylene (Celgard)	Porous	25	-	Very high	Very high
Teflon	Porous	500	-	Very high	Very high

*cc/min, sq m, atm

TABLE III

BLOOD GAS TRANSPORT RATES OF MEMBRANE MATERIALS
UNDER TYPICAL OXYGENATOR CONDITIONS [22]

Material	Construction	Permeation rate*	
		O_2	CO_2**
Silicone rubber	Reinforced with Dacron knit	40 (130)	58
Ultrathin polyfluorinated cellulose	Coated Tyvek	44 (800)	86
Ultrathin PAS	Coated embossed porous polypropylene	52*** (1100)	190
Porous polypropylene (Celgard)	Porous	52*** (high)	270
Teflon	Porous	52*** (high)	250
Gore-Tex	Porous	52*** (high)	260

*cc/min, sq m; under conditions of blood flow and O_2 partial pressure gradient such that a silicone rubber membrane performs as tabulated. All tests with similar cell geometry.

**3 cm Hg ΔP effective driving force for CO_2 transfer.

***Blood film limiting

( )Ideal O_2 transport if membrane limited at 730 torr O_2 pressure.

To test the gas exchange performance of a prototype 0.54 sq m Kolobow spiral coil lung [24] containing an ultrathin polyalkyl-sulfone membrane, we venovenous-perfused an awake lamb for 22 hours. Figure 2 illustrates the oxygen and carbon dioxide transfer rates for this device and compares them to the results published for a similar device containing a supported silicone rubber membrane [25]. While the conditions of the experiments are not identical, comparison is informative because the blood film-limited oxygen rates are closely similar while the polyalkylsulfone membrane permits carbon dioxide transfer rates some five times greater than those measured for a silicone rubber membrane.

BLOOD COMPATIBILITY

The development of blood compatible materials is important to many medical devices including catheters, heart valves, artificial hearts, intraaortic balloon assist devices, blood tubing and other elements of extracorporeal circuits [26]. Only recently have several materials become identified as candidates for materials for membrane lungs, and comparative compatibility testing is necessary.

Earlier animal testing was concerned with minimizing thrombosis and hemorrhage during long-term animal perfusion. Recently, attention has turned to other forms of blood damage, especially thrombocytopenia and platelet injury. Moreover, standard in vitro tests for the thrombotic activity of synthetic surfaces have given contradictory and ambiguous results: at present, surface smoothness and surface purity appear to be two of the most important factors.

Our approach to biocompatibility testing of new materials for membrane artificial lungs has concentrated on ex vivo testing. As an initial screening test, we perform whole blood clotting times using test tubes coated with the test material. Clotting times beyond 20 minutes (standard for siliconized glass) are considered promising. At this point, initial biological testing is performed using several implant tests to rule out local cytotoxicity by long-term intramuscular implantation [27]. Then, if the test material has sufficient strength and gas permeability, it is appropriate to manufacture a simple membrane lung.

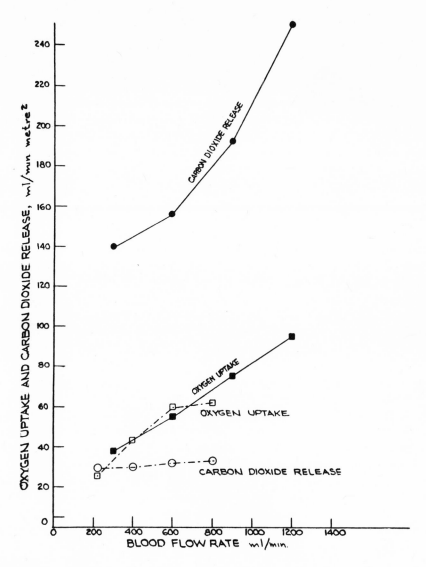

FIGURE 2. Solid line: <u>in vivo</u> venovenous perfusion with 0.54 sq m spiral membrane, PAS on Celgard with Dacron spacer, pH 7.5-7.6, pCO_2 33-36 mm Hg, hematocrit 26%. Dotted line: 0.66 sq m spiral membrane, silicone rubber, pH 7.5, pCO_2 39-42 mm Hg, hematocrit 49%.

Animal Testing - Ex Vivo Methods

For our test system, we utilize prolonged venovenous perfusion of awake, alert lambs as initially described by Kolobow, et al.
[28]. We have found the awake, mildly restrained lamb, eating
and drinking ad lib, to be an ideal model for testing the changes
induced in blood by membrane oxygenators. Lambs (15-25 kg) are
briefly anesthetized and cannulated with thin-walled stainless steel
reinforced segmented polyurethane cannulae (Biomer, Ethicon, Inc.)
[29]. One drainage cannula is placed into the inferior vena cava
via the external jugular vein, another return cannula is placed in
the opposite external jugular vein into the superior vena cava.
Blood is drained via silicone tubing to a silicone reservoir bag,
pumped in a nonocclusive fiberglass reinforced segmented polyurethane (Biomer) pump chamber through an 0.5-1.0 sq m Kolobow
design spiral coil membrane oxygenator and returned through a
cannulating electromagnetic flow probe to the internal jugular vein.
Following cannulation, lambs are allowed to awaken, returned to
a warmed cage and connected to the perfusion system. Lambs are
initially heparinized at 500 units/kg and are then given a heparin
infusion of 80-150 units/kg/hr. The extracorporeal volume is
approximately 400 ml and is primed with Ringer's lactate containing 5,000 units heparin per liter. The extracorporeal perfusion
apparatus is flushed with pure carbon dioxide before priming to
avoid microbubble trapping at irregularities on the membrane [7].
After perfusion, cannulae are removed, the jugular veins are
ligated following reinfusion of the extracorporeal volume and the
animal is returned to his cage. All animals perfused by this technique should be healthy long-term survivors.

Results of Prolonged Ex Vivo Perfusion

Kolobow, et al. reported venovenous bypass using dimethylpolysiloxane membranes filled with 30% silica filler (SSFR) and
standard laboratory silicone tubing [28]. They showed no significant changes in blood proteins, an increase in white cells, and a
small loss of red cells (approximately 3% hematocrit per day)
during week-long bypass. A majority of red cell loss was accounted for by sampling, and bleeding at incision sites, while no
significant free hemoglobin was detectable. Free hemoglobin
levels remained below 10 mg %. However, they noted a significant
fall in blood platelet concentration during extracorporeal perfusion
(Fig. 3). In order to study this platelet destruction, we labeled

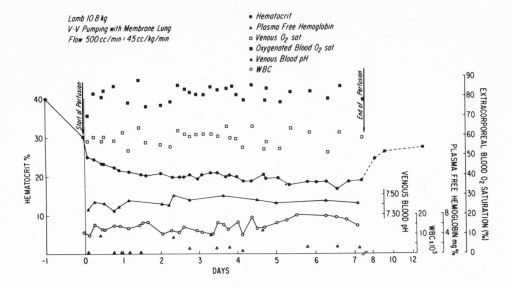

FIGURE 3. One-week venovenous bypass of a 10.8 kg lamb with
an 0.4 sq m spiral coil lung and Biomer chamber nonocclusive
pump. No transfusions given. (Courtesy of Dr. Theodor Kolobow).

lamb platelets with 51-chromium by a modification of the technique
of Aster and Jandl [30]. Autologous labeled platelets were infused and a baseline taken 15-24 hours after infusion. Lambs
were cannulated and perfused for 24 hours during which time blood
samples were taken, platelet rich plasma separated, and the activity of the platelet rich plasma counted. This technique is reported
in a recent paper [31]. A normal unperfused sheep loses 12% of
its circulating platelet radioactivity each day. Our sheep irreversibly lost 50-60% of their blood activity and platelet counts in the
first four hours of perfusion (Fig. 4). We found that drug therapy
did not modify the rate or extent of destruction of platelets as
measured by both platelet count or platelet activity (Figs. 5 and 6).

Recently, Kolobow, et al. described a technique of coating
silicone tubing with 10% pure dimethylpolysiloxane in toluene and
crosslinking this polymer gum with five megarads of high energy
radiation [7]. All connectors are fabricated of stainless steel
and coated with Biomer. We tested this technique in silicone pumping circuits without oxygenators (Figs. 7 and 8) and in combination
with oxygenators whose membrane surfaces were coated with

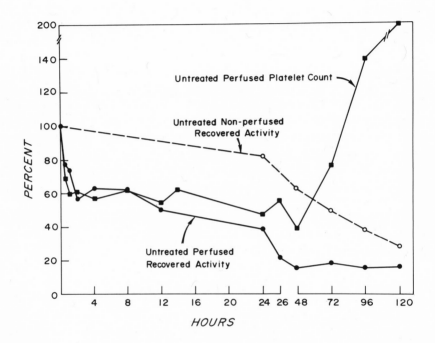

FIGURE 4. The mean blood platelet count for perfused lambs expressed as percent of initial count and corrected for dilution when
applicable. Platelet count for all groups was similar.

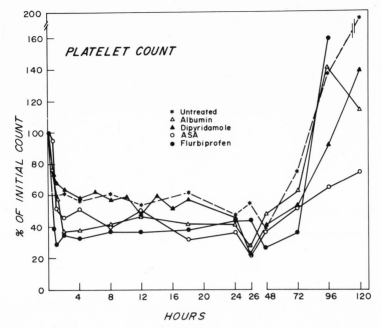

FIGURE 5. The mean platelet count and recovered activity of five untreated perfused (ECP) lambs are compared with recovered radioactivity from untreated nonperfused lambs. Two days after termination of ECP, platelet count rose to 76% of prebypass levels while recovered activity fell to 15-17%.

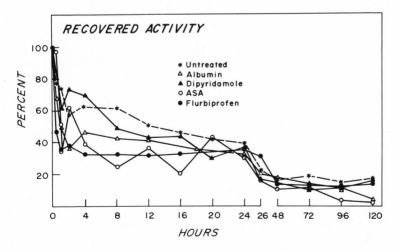

FIGURE 6. Recovered activity during and after 24 hour ECP for perfused lambs. Recovered activity of all groups is similar.

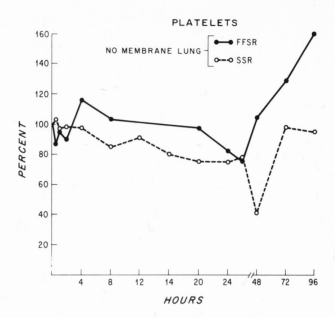

FIGURE 7. Average platelet count (2 lambs in each group) during and after 24 hr venovenous bypass without an oxygenator.

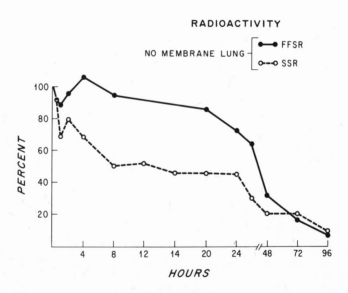

FIGURE 8. Average recovered activity (2 lambs in each group) during and after 24 hr venovenous bypass without an oxygenator.

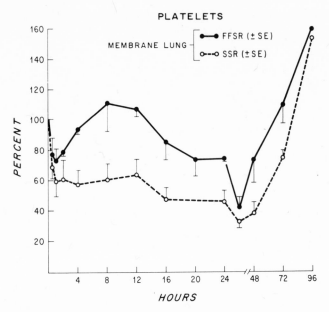

FIGURE 9. Mean blood platelet count during and after 24 hr perfusion with silica-free tubing and oxygenator coatings.

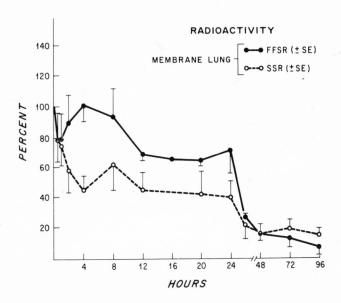

FIGURE 10. Mean recovered activity during and after 24 hr perfusion with silica-free silicone tubing and oxygenator coating.

TABLE IV

ORGAN ^{51}Cr COUNTS FOLLOWING TWO WEEKS
OF CLINICAL PERFUSION FOR ACUTE
RESPIRATORY FAILURE

Tissue	CPM/g tissue	Total organ CPM	% Blood in organ
Heart	14.6	4,380	6
Lungs	55.4	111,222	18
Liver	784	1,881,600	10
Spleen	6,028	1,808,400	36
Blood	173/ml	764,000	100
		4,569,602	

Platelets were labeled 12 hours prior to termination of venovenous perfusion. Silica-filled membrane lung.

silica-free silicone rubber catalyzed by organic peroxide (SFSR)
(Figs. 9 and 10). We have found that there is a significant decrease in destruction and increase in lifespan of platelets exposed to surfaces prepared without silica in this manner.

To illustrate the clinical problem, we labeled homologous
platelets with 51-chromium and infused them during a recent perfusion of a 13-year-old patient with pulmonary failure secondary
to meningococcal septicemia. After two weeks of bypass using a
single 3.5 sq m spiral coil membrane lung containing standard
silica-filled silicone membranes (SSFR), we found extensive platelet destruction and thrombocytopenia (Table IV). Infusion of labeled platelets during venovenous bypass was followed within 12
hours by death of the patient. At autopsy, over 50% of the infused
label was localized in the liver and spleen of the patient. Rapid
destruction of infused platelets with hepatic and splenic sequestration is occurring during clinical prolonged extracorporeal perfusion with standard silica-filled membrane lungs.

Since hemorrhage is a frequent occurrence during extra-corporeal perfusion even at short Lee-White clotting times (<20 min) [2] and thrombocytopenia with hepatic and splenic plate-let sequestration is universal, platelet-sparing membranes are the next phase in membrane lung construction for prolonged per-fusion. We consider this to be a most vital area for research and testing of new generation membrane oxygenators.

Polyalkylsulfone and ethylcellulose perfluorobutyrate mem-brane lungs will be tested for platelet damage during long-term perfusion as these devices are constructed. It is hoped that these new materials will be equally or more effective than silica-free silicone rubber in preventing platelet damage or destruction. Our future goal is prolonged extracorporeal perfusion without heparini-zation, or induced hemostatic defects. At that point, cardio-pulmonary support can be performed in a large group of patients with minimal risk of hemorrhage.

ACKNOWLEDGEMENTS

Supported by NHLI Grant, HL 16154; Contracts HB2916 and HR42919. Dr. Zapol is the recipient of Research Career Develop-ment Award HL70303.

The authors wish to thank Dr. Donald Gray, Dr. James D. Birkett, Ms. Lita Nelsen, Ms. Sheila Bloom and Mr. Thomas Wonders for their assistance.

REFERENCES

1. Hill, J. D., deLeval, M. R., Fallat, R. J., Bramson, M. L., Eberhart, R. C., Schulte, H. D., Osborn, J. J., Barber, R., and Gerbrode, F., J. Thorac. Cardiov. Surg., 64, 551 (1972).

2. Zapol, W. M., Qvist, J., Pontoppidan, H., Liland, A., McEnany, T., and Laver, M. B., ibid., (in press).

3. Gille, J. P., Bull. Physio-Pathol. Respir., 10, 373 (1974).

4. Bellhouse, B. J., Bellhouse, F. H., Curl, C. M., MacMillan, T. I., Gunning, A. J., Spratt, E. H., MacMurray, S. B., and Nelems, J. M., Trans. Amer. Soc. Artif. Intern. Organs, 19, 72 (1973).

5.   Bartlett, R. H., Kittredge, D., Noyes, B. S., Jr., Willard, R. H., III, and Drinker, P. A., J. Thorac. Cardiov. Surg., 58, 795 (1969).

6.   Hill, J. D., Iatridis, A., O'Keefe, R., Kitrilatis, S., Trans. Amer. Soc. Artif. Intern. Organs, 20, 249 (1974).

7.   Kolobow, T., Stool, E. W., Weathersby, P. K., Pierce, J., Hayano, F., and Suaudeau, J., Trans. Amer. Soc. Artif. Intern. Organs, 20, 269 (1974).

8.   Clowes, G.H.A., Hopkins, A. L., and Neville, W. E., J. Thorac. Surg., 32, 630 (1956).

9.   Thomas, J. A., Compt. Rend. Acad Sci., Ser. D, 246, 1084 (1958).

10. Burns, N. and Melrose, D., in Mechanical Devices for Cardiopulmonary Assistance, R. H. Bartlett, P. Drinker, and P. M. Galletti, Eds., Adv. Cardiol., 6, 58 (1971).

11. Kolobow, T. and Spragg, R. G., Med. Instrum., 7, 268 (1973).

12. Dantowitz, P., Borsanyi, A. S., Deibert, M. C., Snider, M. T., Scherler, M., Lipsky, M. H., and Galletti, P. M., Trans. Amer. Soc. Artif. Intern. Organs, 15, 138 (1969).

13. Ketteringham, J. M., Nelsen, L. L., Stevenson, K. K., Birkett, J. D., and Massucco, A. A., Polyalkylsulfones: Blood Compatible Polymers for Membrane Lungs, U. S. Nat. Tech. Info. Serv., Rept. No. NIH-NOI-H8-3-2916-1.

14. Eisman, B., Birnbaum, D., Leonard, R., and Martinez, F. J., Surg., Gynecol., Obstet., 135, 732 (1972).

15. Ketteringham, J. M., Zapol, W. M., Gray, D. N., Stevenson, K. K., Massucco, A. A., Nelsen, L. L., and Cullen, D. P., Trans. Amer. Soc. Artif. Intern. Organs, 19, 61 (1973).

16. Rozelle, L. T., and Petersen, R. J., U. S. Nat. Tech. Inform. Serv., PB Rept. No. 231,324, 1974.

17. Matthews, F. E. and Elder, H. M., British Patent 11,635, (1914).

18. Frederick, D. S., Cogan, H. D., and Marcel, C. S., J. Amer. Chem. Soc., 56, 1815 (1934).

19. Crawford, J. E. and Gray, D. N., J. Appl. Polym. Sci., 15, 1881 (1971).

20. Lautier, A., Bonnet, A., Volter, F., Hung, B. M., and Laurent, D., Trans. Amer. Soc. Artif. Intern. Organs, 20, 307 (1974).

21. Murphy, W., Trudell, L. A., Friedman, L. J., Katvan, M., ibid., 20, 278 (1974).

22. All transfer rates measured in vitro at A.D. Little, Inc., Cambridge, Mass.

23. Marx, T. I., Snyder, W. E., St. John, A. D., Moeller, C. E., J. Appl. Physiol., 15, 1123 (1960).

24. Kolobow, T. and Bowman, R. L., Trans. Amer. Soc. Artif. Intern. Organs, 9, 238 (1963).

25. Kolobow, T. and Zapol, W. M., in Mechanical Devices for Cardiopulmonary Assistance, R. H. Bartlett, P. Drinker, and P. M. Galletti, Eds., Adv. Cardiol., 6, 112 (1971).

26. Bruck, S. D., Blood Compatible Synthetic Polymers: An Introduction, Charles C. Thomas, Springfield, Ill., 1974.

27. Stetson, J. B. and Guess, W. L., Anesthesiology, 33, 635 (1970).

28. Kolobow, T., Zapol, W. M., and Pierce, J., Trans. Amer. Soc. Artif. Intern. Organs, 15, 172 (1969).

29. Kolobow, T. and Zapol, W., Surgery, 68, 625 (1970).

30. Aster, R. H. and Jandl, J. H., J. Clin. Invest., 43, 843 (1964).

31.   Bloom, S., Zapol, W., Wonders, T., Berger, S., and
      Salzman, E., Trans. Amer. Soc. Artif. Intern. Organs,
      20, 299 (1974).

MATERIALS FOR USE IN THE EYE

Miguel F. Refojo

The Retina Foundation, Boston, Massachusetts
02114

Many synthetic polymers and regenerated or chemically modified natural polymers have been used in experimental and clinical ophthalmology. Some areas of this field have been reviewed previously [1, 2, 3, 4, 5]. The most commonly used materials in ophthalmology are poly(methyl methacrylate) (PMMA), silicones, hydrogels, and cyanoacrylate adhesives.

PMMA has often been used in applications requiring its excellent optical properties, such as in contact lenses [6], artificial epithelium [7], artificial corneas [7], and in intracameral lenses [8]. The physicochemical properties of PMMA are well known and will not be discussed in this paper. The safety requirements for ophthalmic use of PMMA can be found in the literature [9].

Silicones also have been widely used in ophthalmology. These polymers have been employed in the eye in the form of oils, particularly in retinal detachment surgery [10]. Silicones have been used to make soft, solid silicone rubber implants for scleral buckling procedures [11], as artificial endothelium [7], as a buried corneal implant [12], and as closed-cell sponges in retinal detachment surgery [13]. Silicones as biomaterials are discussed in this symposium by J. Boretos.

Hydrogels, particularly acrylic hydrogels, were first introduced as biomaterials in ophthalmology [14, 15]. They are mainly used in this field as contact lenses [16]. Hydrogels as biomaterials are discussed in this symposium by A. Hoffman.

Since cyanoacrylate adhesives first became known, considerable attention has been directed to their possible clinical use in
ocular surgery [5]. Due to their availability, bond strength, and
tissue tolerance characteristics, isobutyl and n-butyl cyanoacrylate
adhesives have been preferred in ophthalmology. These adhesives
have been successfully employed as adjuncts to sutures in several
surgical procedures [19]. They have been used to fix prosthetic
devices to the cornea (glued-on contact lenses and penetrating keratoprostheses [17]) and to sclera (sutureless scleral buckling [18]).
However, the uncertain life of the adhesive-tissue bond has limited
the usefulness of these applications. The most favorable clinical
results have been obtained in sealing corneal perforations and lacerations, and in sealing choroidal perforations, e.g., ruptured globes
and leaking pars plana injection sites [19].

Synthetic polymers have been used as medical devices and surgical implants in almost all parts of the eye to improve (contact
and intraocular lenses) or to restore vision (artificial corneas),
for the preservation of sight (scleral buckling materials), as cos-
metic devices to restore the normal appearance of the eye, and in
plastic surgery of tissues surrounding the eye. In this paper we
will briefly review contact lenses, artificial tears, artificial corneas, drainage tubes for treatment of glaucoma, intraocular lenses,
scleral buckling materials, and artificial vitreous substitutes. Excluded from this review will be the suture materials employed in
eye surgery [20], as well as materials used as orbital implants
[21], for socket reconstruction [22], lacrimal canalicular repair
[23], and plastic and reconstructive surgery of the lids [24] and
other tissues surrounding the eye [25].

Contact Lens Materials [6]

The contact lens industry developed rapidly after World War II
with the availability of PMMA. Most hard contact lenses, both
scleral and corneal, are made of PMMA. The high optical quality,
resistance to discoloration, light weight, and excellent molding and
machine qualities of PMMA, as well as its nonirritant nature contributed to the rapid expansion of the contact lens industry.

The corneal surface must be wet and oxygenated at all times
in order to remain transparent and healthy. Normally, tears supply
oxygen from the air to the corneal epithelium. Because PMMA has
very low oxygen permeability (D = 11×10^{-7} sq cm/hr [26]), PMMA

lenses must be fitted so that normal blinking will effect a continuous tear exchange between the lens and the cornea. In addition,
PMMA corneal lenses must float on the tear film in order to avoid
rubbing the corneal epithelium. For optical reasons, contact lenses
must be uniformly wetted on their surface. Although PMMA lenses
absorb moisture up to about 1.5 percent by weight, the PMMA surface is relatively hydrophobic and a wetting adjuvant is often used
with these lenses. Soaking PMMA contact lenses in a wetting solution temporarily improves their wetting properties, but the treatment must be repeated often. To improve the duration of wettability of PMMA lenses, more permanent hydrophilic coatings have
been used [27]. Chemical reactions on the surface layers of the
lens have also been used [28]. However, none of these treatments
have been sufficiently practical, and most hard contact lenses are
still made of unmodified, pure PMMA.

Considering only corneal epithelial oxygenation [29, 30], the
best available synthetic material for contact lenses would be silicone rubber [31, 32] which is highly permeable to oxygen and
carbon dioxide. Unfortunately, silicone rubber is highly hydrophobic and without a hydrophilic coating, either temporary or permanent; contact lenses made of this material are both poor optical
devices and uncomfortable to wear. Surface modification [33] and
wetting solutions can be used to improve silicone contact lenses
[34].

Hydrophilic silicone contact lenses would have two of the most
desirable properties for a contact lens, namely wettability and
oxygen permeability. At least one such contact lens is under investigation. It consists of a graft copolymer of vinyl pyrrolidone
onto an RTV silicone rubber [35].

So far, the main drawback in the availability of any kind of
silicone contact lens appears to be due to manufacturing difficulties,
particularly edging, which is of the utmost importance for comfort
and, ultimately tolerance of corneal contact lenses. However,
clinical testing of some silicone contact lenses is under way, and
there are indications of progress in the manufacture and wettability of such lenses [36].

The pioneer work of Wichterle and Lim [14] over a decade
ago with hydrogels is revolutionizing the contact lens field. The
first hydrogel contact lenses were made from slightly crosslinked
poly(hydroxyethyl methacrylate) (PHEMA), which is still the most

commonly used material for making hydrogel contact lenses. However, because contact lens technology and clinical experience were underdeveloped in Czechoslovakia where these lenses were invented, it was not until PHEMA was brought to the United States, with its advanced contact lens technology and sophisticated contact lens practitioners, that the new and relatively more successful PHEMA hydrogel contact lenses were made available.

Since the introduction of PHEMA contact lenses, there has been a continuous effort to develop other hydrogel contact lenses with improved properties. A variety of hydrogels have been developed, some of which contain HEMA as the main component, while others contain HEMA as only one of a number of principal ingredients.

In addition to HEMA, the second compound most often used as principal ingredient in hydrogel contact lenses has been vinyl pyrrolidone (VP). For example, crosslinked copolymers of VP and HEMA [37], and graft copolymers of HEMA onto PVP [38] have widespread application.

All hydrogel contact lenses are made of sparingly crosslinked polymers, so that the hydrogel lens will have an equilibrium in physiological saline of approximately 40% to 55% H_2O. The most common crosslinking agent, and a minor ingredient in most hydrogel contact lenses, is ethylene glycol dimethacrylate, which is usually present in HEMA monomer as an impurity that is difficult to remove.

The permeability of hydrogel contact lenses to oxygen has been a subject of controversy. Exaggerated claims about the permeability characteristics of most hydrogel lenses have often been made [39]. The opposite view that hydrogel contact lenses are as impermeable to oxygen as hard PMMA contact lenses was also proposed when these lenses first became available [40]. Actually, neither position is correct because hydrogel contact lenses are, in fact, moderately permeable to oxygen. The oxygen flux across hydrogel lenses under physiological conditions is, in most cases, insufficient for normal functioning of the corneal epithelium. However, if the hydrogel lenses are of a certain minimum thickness, sufficient oxygen may permeate through them for normal corneal metabolism [41].

Other hydrogel contact lenses of novel chemical composition have been developed. This is a very active field of investigation, and many new contact lens materials are under investigation. However, the chemical composition of most of these new materials is unfortunately not yet available.

Some new contact lens materials, other than hydrogels and silicones, are under study [42, 43]. These plastic lenses may be somewhat more flexible than PMMA contact lenses, and are said to be highly oxygen permeable.

Ocular Insert Devices for Administration of Drugs

Ocular devices are designed to deliver medication directly to the eye in continuously released and controlled drug dosages. Since drug delivery systems are extensively discussed by other participants of the symposium, ocular drug delivery devices will be only briefly reviewed here. There are essentially three types of ocular insert devices: (1) drug-impregnated insoluble polymers such as hydrogels which will render the drug into the tear film at a variable rate dependent upon the concentration difference; (2) drugs thoroughly mixed with a soluble or biodegradable polymer such as gelatin which will deliver the drug at the rate of degradation or dissolution of the polymer in the tear film; and (3) drugs contained in a reservoir with outside walls made of a permselective polymeric membrane. The rate of transport of a given drug through the membrane can be controlled by the area and thickness of the membrane surrounding the drug reservoir, and by the chemical potential difference across the membrane, i.e., the difference between the reservoir and the tear film. These devices are designed for constant rate release of certain ophthalmic drugs at a predetermined therapeutically effective level [44, 45].

Ocular insert devices are usually circular (about 8 to 10 mm in diameter) or oval-shaped (about 8 x 4 mm) flat discs which are inserted and maintained under the lower eyelid for variable lengths of time. The interval of constant release usually ranges between 24 hours and one week, depending on the medication. These devices are soft and hydrophilic and, after a short time, patients are not aware of their presence in the eye [46].

The instillation of eye drops supplies peak doses of a drug, usually at levels higher than required. The dosage decreases rapidly to below therapeutic levels until the next drop is instilled. This disadvantage is overcome by ocular insert devices which continuously release a drug into the tear film at a set rate and maintain the appropriate dosage until the device is replaced.

A similar mechanism of continuous drug delivery is provided by drug-impregnated hydrogel contact lenses [47, 48]. The nature of the drug, the concentration of the impregnating solution, the nature of polymer matrix, and the size and thickness of the impregnated lens combine to determine the dosage supplied to the eye. The drug delivery rate, however, is subject to some variation. The main difference between an impregnated hydrogel contact lens and an ocular insert device is that the contact lens delivers the drug directly to the whole cornea as well as to the tear film, while the ocular insert device delivers the drug only to the tear film and directly to small portions of the conjunctiva.

The continuous delivery of drugs to a target organ is a controversial topic and some investigators still believe that pulse delivery may be more effective therapeutically than continuous delivery of smaller doses. In addition, there has been some fear of cumulative toxicity from the continuous delivery system. More time is needed to determine if ocular insert devices, which now appear highly desirable to most investigators, will become routine therapeutical devices.

Polymers in Artificial Tears

In some dry eye conditions, and in certain solutions to be used with contact lenses, artificial tears are required. An isotonic sodium chloride solution and similar buffered salt solutions are very useful for these cases, but they have a relatively short retention time in the eye. To avoid frequent instillation of drops, a variety of water soluble polymers have been dissolved in artificial tear solutions and in other ophthalmic preparations. The polymers increase the viscosity and the retention time of the wetting solution in the eye, but increased viscosity is probably not the only contributing effect of the polymers [49]. Some of these solutions are very useful clinically. Among the polymers employed in ophthalmic solutions are methylcellulose and other cellulose derivatives such as hydroxypropylcellulose, polyvinyl alcohol, polyvinyl pyrrolidone, and polyethylene glycol [50, 51].

Artificial Corneas

There are at least as many models of keratoprostheses and as many procedures of prosthokeratoplasty as there are investigators interested in this problem [52]. Cardona, the most active investigator in this field, has worked on as many as twelve different types of keratoprostheses [53]. However, all the penetrating keratoprostheses are essentially of one of two designs, the collar-button shaped prosthesis which sandwiches the cornea between two plastic plates [54], and the prosthesis with an intracorneal supporting flange [55].

Most keratoprostheses are made of PMMA. Sometimes only the optical portion of the prosthesis, a cylinder of variable dimensions from the anterior chamber to the corneal surface, is made of PMMA. The cylinder supporting flange or skirt may be made of Dacron, Teflon, nylon or a similar biocompatible porous material [56].

Through the years, investigators have attempted to obtain a sound biological attachment between the corneal tissue and keratoprostheses. Stone, et al. [55] used fenestrations in the intralamellar skirt of the prosthesis through which fibrous tissue can grow. Girard, et al. [57] obtained fixation with a skirt of Dacron mesh, similar to the one devised by Cardona, who used a skirt of siliconized Teflon [56].

An interesting solution to this problem was devised by Strampelli [58]. His odontokeratoprosthesis consists of an optical plastic inlay with a flange of autogenous bone and dentine. The bone portion of the flange is located anteriorly and is covered with a labial mucosa in the cornea. The dentine is posteriorly located, lying over the recipient cornea. The adherence of the host tissue to the prosthesis occurs by infiltration of the bone with fibrous tissue.

While several types of keratoprostheses have been successful in selected patients, a generally accepted keratoprosthesis is not yet available. Particularly unfortunate is the fact that the patients who could benefit the most from prosthokeratoplasty have the highest rate of failure [59].

Artificial Epithelium

In some corneal diseases, the irregularity of the anterior layer of the cornea, the epithelium, is the cause of poor vision. It has been possible to replace the corneal epithelium with a PMMA contact lens glued with a cyanoacrylate adhesive to the collagen tissue that underlies the corneal epithelium [60]. The glued-on contact lenses are termed epikeratoprostheses [61]. In most instances, this procedure is initially well-tolerated, but the adhesive-tissue bond often fails after a period of a few weeks to a few months. Epithelium will then grow under the lens with subsequent irritation, requiring its removal [62].

Fluid Barrier Procedures

Edema of the corneal epithelium is caused by the accumulation of fluid flowing in an anterior direction due to a deficient endothelium. It was, therefore, postulated that a fluid-impermeable membrane or prosthesis in or behind the cornea would reduce corneal edema anterior to it [7]. Three types of fluid barriers have been used: (1) intralamellar membranes, usually PMMA discs sandwiched in the cornea [63]; (2) buried mushroom-shaped implants made of PMMA [64] or silicone rubber [65]; and (3) artificial endothelium, which is created by attaching a silicone membrane to the posterior part of the cornea [66]. The usefulness of fluid barrier procedures is limited by the fact that the membranes and implants are not only a barrier to fluids but also to the nutrients that the anterior portions of the cornea normally receive from the anterior chamber [7]. After several months, or even years, some of the patients with fluid barrier membranes or implants develop degeneration of the corneal tissue anterior to the implant.

Eye Drainage Procedures in Glaucoma

Glaucoma is a condition marked by increase in intraocular pressure, which, if untreated, leads to blindness. When glaucoma does not respond to more conservative modalities of treatment, tubes are implanted to drain aqueous humor and alleviate the excessive pressure [67, 68, 69]. Usually, one end of the tube is placed in the anterior chamber of the eye and the other end drains the aqueous humor into the subconjunctival or suprachoroidal spaces. Unfortunately, the reduction in pressure in most glaucomatous eyes operated in this way is only temporary. The ultimate reason for failure is usually the occlusion of the tube to fibrous proliferation around the end of the tube in the subconjunctival or suprachoroidal spaces.

To eliminate this difficulty, Lee and Schepens [70] investigated a drainage system between the anterior chamber and an extraocular vein. Because the intraocular pressure is higher than the extraocular venous pressure, unidirectional flow of aqueous humor into the vein takes place, and the intraocular pressure decreases. The failures with this method have been attributed to slippage of the capillary tube from the vein, venous thrombosis, and blood clots in the tube. Among the many materials used for the drainage procedure, the most common are polyethylene and silicone rubber. Reconstituted collagen is currently being investigated in the aqueous-venous shunt of Lee.

Intraocular Lenses

Intraocular lenses are sometimes used to correct visual function following cataract surgery [71]. These lenses can be anterior chamber implants or posterior chamber implants [72]. Intraocular lenses are most commonly made of PMMA, sometimes with nylon fixation loops. Normally, failure of artificial lenses is due to surgical or mechanical factors and not to material toxicity. Since the implantation of intraocular lenses can have serious complications, this procedure should be performed only when a contact lens cannot provide the same level of visual acuity [73].

Scleral Buckling Materials

When the retina separates from the wall of the eye because of traction exerted by vitreous structures, trauma, or as a result of pathological conditions, it loses contact with its source of nutrition, the blood vessels of the choroid. Retinal detachment, if left untreated, causes blindness. Traction on the retina can be counteracted by indenting the wall of the eye from the outside in the area of the retinal break.

Several absorbable and nonabsorbable scleral implants have been used in retinal detachment surgery to produce a buckling effect. Implants made of materials that swell postoperatively, such as absorbable gelatin [74] or a nonabsorbable material such as poly(glyceryl methacrylate) hydrogel [75], can be used to produce scleral buckles. However, full indentation is somewhat delayed by the gradual swelling process.

Polyethylene tubing was the material of choice for several years, but its rigidity caused erosion of the eye walls [76]. Solid, soft silicone rubber [77] and closed-cell type silicone sponges [13] are now commonly used in scleral buckling operations. Both types of materials have their supporters.

A new type of expandable silicone rubber implant has recently been developed [78]. The main advantage of this type of implant is that the size of the scleral buckling can be easily modified during or after surgery by injecting fluid into the implant.

The incidence of infection after retinal detachment surgery using scleral buckling materials is relatively low. When meticulous, sterile procedures are followed, approximately two percent of the operated cases develop infection. Infection has been attributed to such diverse factors as the duration of the operative procedure, the nature and physical form of the material used to create the buckle (i.e., solid silicone or silicone sponges), and the impediment to fluid exchange between the treated tissue and its surroundings created by the implant. In addition, the persistence of bacteria in the area of the implant, despite scrupulously aseptic conditions, has been demonstrated in over half the cases studied [79, 80]. The incidence of infection can be reduced by the sustained release of antibiotics from materials used to produce scleral buckling [81].

Gelatin and other hydrogel implants readily absorb aqueous solutions of antibiotics. Their antibacterial potency depends upon the size of the implant, the type of antibiotic used, and the duration of treatment. The antibacterial activity of gelatin and acrylic hydrogel implants dipped in solutions of lincomycin and chloramphenicol decreased rapidly, and was lost after only three or four days of elution [81].

Chloramphenicol sodium succinate and lincomycin hydrochloride can be successfully incorporated into solid silicone rubber and into closed-cell silicone sponges by using propylene oxide as a vehicle. This solvent is removed by evaporation, leaving the antibiotics trapped in the implants. Solid antibiotics can also be compounded into solid silicone rubber implants prior to vulcanization at room temperature [81].

Artificial Vitreous

In some complex cases of retinal detachment, it is useful to supplement, expand, or replace the vitreous humor of the eye [82]. Absorbable and nonabsorbable substances have been employed for this purpose [83]. Absorbable materials, such as physiological saline and air, are replaced gradually by newly secreted intra-ocular fluids. Silicone oil, a nonabsorbable substance, has been injected into the vitreous cavity as an adjunct to scleral buckling and other retinal detachment procedures [10, 84]. This procedure has been used quite often. However, improvement of vision with silicone was temporary and visual deterioration ensued as a consequence of retinal degeneration [85].

The search for an ideal vitreous substitute continues. There is a need for a material which will tamponade the retina against the choroid during the formation of chorioretinal adhesion, but will not pass through a retinal break. Disregarding for the moment the physiological problems inherent in the use of any substitute, the physical properties and methods of introducing vitreous substitutes into the eye will now be discussed.

Gases [86] and low viscosity liquids can penetrate a retinal break and their usefulness as vitreous substitutes is thus limited. Liquids of high viscosity are less likely to penetrate through retinal holes. The ideal physical properties for a vitreous substitute are those of a gel similar to the natural vitreous body of the eye. Such a substitute must be introduced into the eye with as little trauma as possible. It would therefore be preferable to inject a vitreous substitute with a needle through the wall of the eye, rather than to introduce it through a surgical incision.

A liquid substance which will gel immediately upon injection into the eye would be ideal. Some viscous polymer solutions become gels after standing undisturbed or after cooling. These gels, which can be liquified again under shear stress (as for example, when the gel is forced through a narrow needle), are known as thixotropic gels. None of these, as far as we know, have been used as vitreous substitutes.

Hyaluronic acid preparations form very thick elastoviscous bodies, particularly at a nonphysiologic, low pH such as 2.5. These differ from true gels in that they retain the flowing and mixing characteristics of liquid, for true gels behave like solids. A true gel

will not flow, nor will two pieces of a broken gel spontaneously
fuse [87]. The reaction of the eye to hyaluronic acid is not consistently good [88]. Each batch of hyaluronic acid must be tested
in experimental animals to ascertain its effect before it can be
used in a vitreous injection.

Irreversible gels crosslinked by primary bonds, such as biodegradable collagen gels [89] and nonbiodegradable acrylic gels
[90], have been used as vitreous substitutes in experimental animals and in a limited number of patients [91]. In a recent report
on the use of collagen gel as vitreous substitute, it was concluded
that the gel cannot be injected into the eye without breaking into
several pieces [92]. Intactness of an implanted vitreous gel is
essential not only for adequate tamponade, but also to insure that
no fragments penetrate behind the detached retina. Moreover,
optical considerations require that an implant be intact. A frag-
mented gel in the vitreous cavity creates a visual impediment.
The larger the number of gel fragments, the higher the scatter of
light, and consequently, the lower the transparency of the media
[93].

If a gel is to be injected into the eye and not pass through retinal breaks or hinder vision by undue scattering of light, it must be
prepared in a suitable injecting device, preferably tubular in shape
with a gradually narrowing funnel-like end connected to the injection needle. A cylindrical vitreous implant of a highly hydrated
gel injected in this manner is very soft and can easily completely
fill the vitreous cavity.

A permanent vitreous implant which could be used in the man-
agement of complex cases of retinal detachment should have the
following properties: (1) it must tamponade the retina against the
choroid and give continuous support to the detached retina; (2) it
must counteract traction exerted by preretinal organization without
causing the formation of additional vitreoretinal adhesions; (3) the
material should be biologically inert and should have a specific
gravity, refractive index, and rigidity approximating that of the
natural gel; (4) it must not hinder transportation of metabolites inside the vitreous cavity. Poly(glyceryl methacrylate) hydrogel of
about 98 percent water by weight at equilibrium in physiological
saline has been used as a vitreous implant [90]. The dehydrated
gel is placed in the vitreous cavity through a small incision in the
pars plana ciliaris. Inside the eye, the implant swells by absorbing injected saline and available intraocular fluids. The final

volume of the gel, i.e., its equilibrium swelling, is known prior
to injection [94, 95].   The softness of these hydrogels approxi-
mates that of the vitreous body.   PGMA hydrogels are well
tolerated by ocular tissues.   However, the principal drawback of
these implants is the relatively slow rate of swelling.   The final
size of the vitreous implant is not reached during the operation
but several hours later.

An intravitreous silicone balloon was designed for cases of
retinal detachment considered inoperable by the current surgical
techniques of scleral buckling, vitreous injection, and vitreous
surgery.   The balloon consists of silicone sheets 0.1 mm thick,
glued together with a silicone adhesive.   A silicone tube, 0.6 mm
outer diameter, is inserted between the sheets to provide an open-
ing for expansion of the balloon.   When filled with physiological
saline, the balloon becomes transparent.   It is introduced into the
vitreous cavity through an incision in the pars plana ciliaris.   The
balloon is expanded inside the vitreous cavity, and the filling tube
is closed, sutured to the sclera, and covered by the conjunctiva.
The intravitreous balloon was designed for use as a temporary implant that would tamponade the retina.   It can be removed at a later
date [96].

ACKNOWLEDGEMENT

Supported by PHS Grant EY-00327 of the National Eye Institute,
National Institutes of Health.

REFERENCES

1. Stone, W., Jr., N. Engl. J. Med., 258, 486-92, 533-40,
    596-602 (1958).

2. Lieb, W. A., Geeraets, W. J., Guerry, D., III, and
    Dickerson, T., Eye, Ear, Nose, Throat Mon., 38, 210, 303
    (1959).

3. Dohlman, C. H. and Freeman, H. M., Doc. Ophthalmol.,
    25, 1 (1968).

4. Refojo, M. F., J. Biomed. Mater. Res., 5, 113 (1971).

5.   Refojo, M. F., Dohlman, C. H., and Koliopoulos, J., Surv.
     Ophthalmol., 15, 217 (1971).

6.   Refojo, M. F., in The Preocular Tear Film and Dry Eye
     Syndromes, F. J. Holly and M. A. Lemp, Eds., Int.
     Ophthalmol. Clin., 13, 263 (1973).

7.   Dohlman, C. H. and Refojo, M. F., in Corneal Edema,
     C. H. Dohlman, Ed., Int. Ophthalmol. Clin., 8, 729 (1968).

8.   Choyce, D. P., Ann. Ophthalmol., 5, 1113 (1973).

9.   Estevez, J.M.J. and Ridley, F., Amer. J. Ophthalmol.,
     62, 132 (1966).

10. Cockerman, W., Schepens, C. L., and Freeman, H. M.,
     Mod. Probl. Ophthalmol., 8, 525 (1969).

11. Schepens, C. L. and Freeman, H. M., in Modern Trends
     in Ophthalmology, A. Sorby, Ed., Vol. 4, Butterworths,
     London, 1967, p. 209.

12. Brown, S. I. and Dohlman, C. H., Arch. Ophthalmol., 73,
     635 (1965).

13. Lincoff, H. A., Baras, I., and McLean, J., ibid., 73, 160
     (1965).

14. Wichterle, O. and Lim, D., Nature, 185, 117 (1960).

15. Wichterle, O. and Lim, D., U. S. Patent 3, 220, 960 (1965).

16. Refojo, M. F., Surv. Ophthalmol., 16, 233 (1972).

17. Dohlman, C. H., Refojo, M. F., Webster, R. G., and
     Richards, J.S.F., Excerpta Medica Int. Cong. Ser. No. 222,
     Ophthalmol., Proc. 21st Int. Cong., 1970, p. 1292.

18. Calabria, G. A., Pruett, R. C., and Refojo, M. F., Arch.
     Ophthalmol., 86, 82 (1971).

19. Webster, R. G., Jr. and Refojo, M. F., in Tissue Adhesives
     in Surgery, T. Matsumoto, Ed., Medical Examination Pub-
     lishing Co., Inc., Flushing, N. Y., 1972, p. 316.

20. Partridge, J., Rich, A., Dunlap, W., and McPherson, S. D., Arch. Ophthalmol., 90, 271 (1973).

21. Browning, C. W., Amer. J. Ophthalmol., 63, 955 (1967).

22. Dortzbach, R. K. and Callahan, A., ibid., 70, 800 (1970).

23. Keith, C. G., ibid., 65, 70 (1968).

24. Banuelos, A., Arch. Ophthalmol., 89, 329 (1973).

25. Dunlap, E. A., Trans. Amer. Ophthalmol. Soc., 65, 393 (1967).

26. Shaw, G., Trans. Faraday Soc., 63, 2181 (1967).

27. Koven, A. L., Eye, Ear, Nose, Throat Mon., 41, 47 (1962).

28. Deaton, J. M. and Hodkins, J. E., Tex. J. Sci., 17, 125 (1965).

29. Hill, R. M. and Schoessler, J., J. Amer. Optom. Assoc., 38, 480 (1967).

30. Burns, R. P., Roberts, H., and Rich, L. F., Amer. J. Ophthalmol., 71, 486 (1971).

31. Becker, W. E., U. S. Patent 3,228,741 (1962).

32. Burdick, D. F., Mishler, J. L., and Polmanteer, K. E., U. S. Patent 3,341,490 (1967).

33. Feneberg, P. and Krekeler, U., German Patent 2,165,905 (1973).

34. Breger, J. L., Optician, 162, 12 (1971).

35. Laizier, J. and Wajs, G., U. S. Patent 3,700,573 (1972).

36. Zekman, T. N. and Sarnat, L. A., Amer. J. Ophthalmol., 74, 534 (1972).

37. Seiderman, M., U. S. Patent 3,721,657 (1973).

38.   O'Driscoll, K. F. and Isey, A. A., U. S. Patent 3,700,761, (1972).

39.   Morrison, D. R. and Edelhauser, H. F., Invest. Ophthalmol., 11, 58 (1972).

40.   Takahashi, G. H., Goldstick, T. K., and Fatt, I., Brit. Med. J., 1, 142 (1966).

41.   Holly, F. J. and Refojo, M. F., J. Amer. Optom. Assoc., 43, 1173 (1972).

42.   Stahl, N. O., Reich, L. A., and Ivani, E., ibid., 45, 302 (1974).

43.   Kamath, P. K., U. S. Patent 3,551,035 (1970).

44.   Pavan-Langston, D., in The Preocular Tear Film and Dry Eye Syndromes, F. J. Holly and M. A. Lemp, Eds., Int. Ophthalmol. Clin., 13, 231 (1973).

45.   Michaels, A. S., Amer. Chem. Soc., Div. Org. Coat. Plast. Chem. Prepr., 34, 559 (1974).

46.   Dohlman, C. H., Pavan-Langston, D., and Rose, J., Ann. Ophthalmol., 4, 823 (1972).

47.   Podos, S. M., Becker, B., Asseff, C., and Hartstein, J., Amer. J. Ophthalmol., 73, 336 (1972).

48.   Maddox, Y. T. and Berstein, H. N., Ann. Ophthalmol., 4, 789 (1972).

49.   Lemp, M. A., in The Preocular Tear Film and Dry Eye Syndromes, F. J. Holly and M. A. Lemp, Eds., Int. Ophthalmol. Clin., 13, 221 (1973).

50.   Lemp, M. A. and Holly, F., Ann. Ophthalmol., 4, 15 (1972).

51.   Rankin, B. F., U. S. Patent 3,755,561 (1973).

52.   Day, R., Trans. Amer. Ophthalmol. Soc., 55, 455 (1957).

53.   Polack, F. M., in Corneal and External Diseases of the Eye,
      Charles C. Thomas, Springfield, Ill., Chapter 37, 1970, p. 319.

54.   Dohlman, C. H., Webster, R. G., Biswas, S. K., and
      Refojo, M. F., Arch. Ophthalmol. (Paris), 29, 169 (1969).

55.   Stone, W., Jr., Yasuda, H., and Refojo, M. F., in The
      Cornea - World Congress, J. H. King and J. W. McTigue,
      Eds., Butterworths, Reading, Mass., 1965, p. 654.

56.   Cardona, H., Amer. J. Ophthalmol., 64, 228 (1967).

57.   Girard, L. J., Moore, C. D., Soper, J. W., and O'Bannon,
      W., Trans. Amer. Acad. Ophthalmol. Otolaryngol., 73,
      936 (1969).

58.   Strampelli, B. and Marchi, V., Ann. Ottal., 96, 1 (1970).

59.   Polack, F. M., Brit. J. Ophthalmol., 55, 838 (1971).

60.   Dohlman, C. H., Carroll, J. M., Ahmad, B., and Refojo,
      M. F., Trans. Amer. Acad. Ophthalmol. Otolaryngol.,
      73, 482 (1969).

61.   Kaufman, H. E. and Gasset, A. R., Amer. J. Ophthalmol.,
      67, 38 (1969).

62.   Dohlman, C. H., Carroll, J. M., Richards, J., and Refojo,
      M. F., Arch. Ophthalmol., 83, 10 (1970).

63.   Choyce, P., Brit. J. Ophthalmol., 49, 432 (1965).

64.   Castroviejo, R., Cardona, H., and DeVoe, A. G., Amer.
      J. Ophthalmol., 68, 613 (1969).

65.   Brown, S. I. and Dohlman, C. H., Arch. Ophthalmol., 73,
      635 (1965).

66.   Dohlman, C. H. and Dubé, I., ibid., 79, 150 (1968).

67.   Ellis, R. A., Amer. J. Ophthalmol., 50, 733 (1960).

68.   Ore, S., Sebestyen, J. G., and Stone, W., Jr., Surgery,
      52, 385 (1962).

69.   Lee, P. F. and Schepens, C. L., Invest. Ophthalmol., $\underline{5}$, 304 (1966).

70.   Lee, P. F. and Schepens, C. L., ibid., $\underline{5}$, 59 (1966).

71.   Jaffe, N. S., Eye, Ear, Nose, Throat Mon., $\underline{51}$, 290 (1972).

72.   Choyce, D. P., Ann. Ophthalmol., $\underline{5}$, 1113 (1973).

73.   van Balen, A.T.M., Amer. J. Ophthalmol., $\underline{75}$, 755 (1973).

74.   Daniele, S., Jacklin, N. H., Schepens, C. L., and Freeman, H. M., Arch. Ophthalmol., $\underline{80}$, 115 (1968).

75.   Calabria, G. A., Pruett, R. C., and Refojo, M. F., ibid., $\underline{86}$, 77 (1971).

76.   Regan, C.D.J. and Schepens, C. L., Trans. Amer. Acad. Ophthalmol. Otolaryngol., $\underline{67}$, 335 (1963).

77.   Schepens, C. L. and Freeman, H. M., in Modern Trends in Ophthalmology, A. Sorsby, Ed., Butterworths, London, 1967, p. 209.

78.   Banuelos, A., Refojo, M. F., and Schepens, C. L., Arch. Ophthalmol., $\underline{89}$, 500 (1973).

79.   McMeel, J. W., ibid., $\underline{74}$, 45 (1965).

80.   Lincoff, H. A., McLean, J. M., and Nano, H., ibid., $\underline{74}$, 641 (1965).

81.   Refojo, M. F., and Thomas, D. A., Ophthalmol. Res. (in press).

82.   Peyman, G. A., Ericson, E. S., and May, D. R., Surv. Ophthalmol. $\underline{17}$, 41 (1972).

83.   Gombos, G. M. and Berman, E. R., Acta Ophthalmol. $\underline{45}$, 794 (1967).

84.   Okun, E., Trans. Pac. Coast Oto-Ophthalmol. Soc., $\underline{49}$, 141 (1968).

85.   Lee, P. F., Donovan, R. H., Mukai, N., et al., Ann.
      Ophthalmol., 1, 15 (1969).

86.   Vygantas, C. M., Peyman, G. A., Daily, M. J., and
      Ericson, E. S., Arch. Ophthalmol., 90, 235 (1973).

87.   Balazs, E. A., Freeman, M. I., Klöti, R., et al., Mod.
      Probl. Ophthalmol., 10, 3 (1972).

88.   Constable, I. J. and Swann, D. S., Arch. Ophthalmol., 88,
      544 (1972).

89.   Dunn, M. W., Stenzel, K. H., Rubin, A. L., et al., ibid.,
      82, 840 (1969).

90.   Daniele, S., Refojo, M. F., Schepens, C. L., and Freeman,
      H. M., ibid., 80, 120 (1968).

91.   Dunn, M., Shafer, D., Stenzel, K. H., et al., Trans Amer.
      Soc. Artif. Intern. Organs, 17, 421 (1971).

92.   Pruett, R. C., Schepens, C. L., and Freeman, H. M.,
      Arch. Ophthalmol., 91, 29 (1974).

93.   Refojo, M. F. and Zauberman, H., Invest. Ophthalmol.,
      12, 465 (1973).

94.   Refojo, M. F., J. Biomed. Mater. Res. Symp. No. 1, 179
      (1971).

95.   Refojo, M. F., An. Quim., 68, 697 (1972).

96.   Tolentino, F. I., Liu, H. S., Refojo, M. F., and Freeman,
      H. M., Annual Meeting of the Association for Research in
      Vision and Ophthalmology, Sarasota, Fla., May 3-7, 1973,
      p. 30.

INDEX